PRAISE FOR *YOUR MONEY OR YOUR LIFE*

"The German word for debt is the same word for guilt. But you don't have to be German to be a guilty debtor in the United States, where the sin of being ill and poor is discharged by indentured labor and the harassment of the debt collector. Luke Messac takes us on a tour of the underbelly of America's hospitals and their horrific debt practices. If there's one country where you don't want to be both poor and ill, it's the United States."
—**Mark Blyth**, The William R. Rhodes '57
Professor of International Economics, The Watson Institute
for International and Public Affairs, Brown University

"A crystal-clear critique of the travesty of profit-driven US medicine by a historian drawing on archives, oral history, public records, and his own ethnographic experience as a doctor delivering emergency care medicine for a typically predatory 'non-profit hospital' that bankrupts its poorest, most vulnerable patients. All medical students should read this book to prevent themselves from inadvertently becoming cogs in a monstrous wheel that indebts their lowest income patients."
—**Philippe Bourgois**, Author, *In Search of Respect:*
Selling Crack in El Barrio and Co-Author, *Righteous Dopefiend*

"In the wake of the COVID-19 pandemic, the impetus for transforming the American health care system is more urgent than ever. Doctor and historian Luke Messac shows how the system has been warped by growing financialization and profiteering, with disastrous consequences for the millions of people struggling with medical debt. Both infuriating and illuminating, he paints a portrait too compelling to ignore."
—**Dave A. Chokshi**, 43rd Health Commissioner of New York City

"*Your Money or Your Life* offers a rare, deeply powerful, and impressively original look at the roots of medical greed and how and why health care debt is driving down the health of our nation. This book is a passionate and inspiring expression of the importance of empowering community leaders and residents to advocate for affordable, accessible, and equitable health care before it's too late. It provides the roadmap, now it's up to all of us to heed the charge."

—**Daniel E. Dawes**, Author, *The Political Determinants of Health*

"Usually, doctors keep themselves aloof from their patients' financial troubles, but not Luke Messac. *Your Money or Your Life* shows how medical debt and the fear of debt decimate family finances and prevent sick people from seeking needed care. Dr. Messac, a historian and emergency physician, is one of our most important critics of the US health system. His voice is engaging and compassionate, and we must listen."

—**Beatrix Hoffman**, Professor of History, Northern Illinois University and Author, *The Wages of Sickness* and *Health Care for Some*

"In *Your Money or Your Life*, Luke Messac weaves together the compelling, and true, story of how medical debt collection became so aggressive and its real-world impact. Taking readers on a remarkable—and eminently readable—journey through the history and practice of medical debt collection, Luke Messac offers the definitive documentation of how deeply embedded medical debt collection practices are to health care finance in America. You will learn about senior citizens doing hard labor to pay off hospital bills, patients getting jailed for missing a court date about their late medical bills, and hospitals foreclosing on homes when former patients fall behind on medical bill payment. Ultimately, this great book demonstrates how these events are not aberrations or one-off errors in judgment, but baked into the design of American health care and the institutions that profit from the sidelines. Dr. Messac's book proves that it will take more than occasional finger wagging or modest reforms around the edges to ensure that patients and doctors are no longer debtors and creditors. Everyone, and I do mean everyone, should read *Your Money or Your Life*."

—**Melissa B. Jacoby**, Graham Kenan Professor of Law, University of North Carolina at Chapel Hill

"In *Your Money or Your Life*, Dr. Messac provides a piercing and must-read investigation into how medical debt came to be such a powerful and grim force in American medicine. To create change for the millions of American families beset by the financial toxicity of our health care system, we must learn from this difficult history."

—**Victor Roy**, Physician, Sociologist, and Author, *Capitalizing a Cure: How Finance Controls the Price and Value of Medicines*

Your Money or Your Life

Debt Collection in American Medicine

Luke Messac

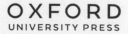

OXFORD
UNIVERSITY PRESS

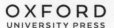

OXFORD
UNIVERSITY PRESS

Oxford University Press is a department of the University of Oxford. It furthers
the University's objective of excellence in research, scholarship, and education
by publishing worldwide. Oxford is a registered trade mark of Oxford University
Press in the UK and certain other countries.

Published in the United States of America by Oxford University Press
198 Madison Avenue, New York, NY 10016, United States of America.

Library of Congress Cataloging-in-Publication Data
Names: Messac, Luke, author.
Title: Your money or your life : debt collection in American medicine /
   Luke Messac.
Description: New York : Oxford University Press, [2024] |
   Includes bibliographical references and index.
Identifiers: LCCN 2023017233 (print) | LCCN 2023017234 (ebook) |
   ISBN 9780197676639 (hardback) | ISBN 9780197676653 (epub) |
   ISBN 9780197676660
Subjects: MESH: Patient Credit and Collection | Accounts Payable and
   Receivable | United States
Classification: LCC RA410.53 (print) | LCC RA410.53 (ebook) | NLM W 80 |
   DDC 338.4/73621—dc23/eng/20230721
LC record available at https://lccn.loc.gov/2023017233
LC ebook record available at https://lccn.loc.gov/2023017234

DOI: 10.1093/oso/9780197676639.001.0001

Printed by Sheridan Books, Inc., United States of America

To my parents, who inspired me to work to build the future,
and to my daughter, Madeleine, who gives me a reason to keep trying.

CONTENTS

ACKNOWLEDGMENTS

I began this book out of a sense of betrayal. Medicine, I thought, is not what it should be, what it can be. I wanted to know why. But in researching and writing this history, I benefited from the loyalty, friendship, and guidance of so many.

As always, librarians proved ever-ready sources of information and hidden treasures, leading me through paywalls and mining old records. Sue Warthman at Brigham and Women's Hospital and the librarians at Rockefeller Library at Brown University were patient, knowledgeable, and resourceful.

My editor, Sarah Humphreville, helped me think through my ideas for the book and hone the tone, style, and argument. She has always been an advocate for my work within the Press. Her editorial colleague, Emma Hodgdon, also provided incisive comments on the manuscript.

Mary Lederer helped with copy editing, citations, and indexing, and was always ready with words of encouragement. I am so grateful for the people who took time to read the book proposal and early drafts, including Mark Blyth, Shay Strauss, Jason Chernesky, Imani Fonfield, and Paula McNulty (who also merits far more thanks for being my mom). Courtney Petrouski and Mat Budelman are amazing friends and offered some great design ideas, one of which was the basis for the cover. Jason Silverstein and the team at *Peste* allowed me to publish part of Chapter 3 in their (absolutely essential) online publication in 2022. I also benefited from conversations and questions at presentations I gave at conferences and on grand rounds, at the University of Nevada Las Vegas Department of Emergency Medicine, the Brown University Department of Emergency Medicine, and the 2022 National Conference for Physician-Scholars in the Social Sciences and Humanities at UCLA.

When I questioned my own hospital's use of lawsuits to collect debts from poor patients, I was not a favorite among C-suite executives, but I had the steadfast support and guidance of my fellow residents, mentors, and program directors, who I am pretty sure do not want to be mentioned by name. But I hope they know how deeply indebted I am to them.

I never would have been able to start down the path of the history of medicine without the patient mentorship of Robert Aronowitz and Steven Feierman. I am also a grateful student of many expert teachers, including Deborah Boucoyannis, Thomas Ponniah, David Barnes, Philippe Bourgois, and Projit Mukharji. My old and new homes, the Rhode Island Hospital and Brigham and Women's Hospital Departments of Emergency Medicine, have been great places to research and write about the past, present, and future of medicine. The doctors, nurses, techs, and staff there taught me how to care for patients with as much skill and compassion as our broken system allows.

My wife, Jamie, the most caring and conscientious doctor I know, shared her thoughts on the horrors of medical debt even as she worked to care for patients amidst the horrors of a pandemic. Her family is filled with medical professionals; her mother, Cathy, was a nurse, and her father, James, a doctor. Both of her sisters, Melanie and Samantha, are physicians. Melanie's daughters, Nina and Josie, are more than comfortable with the medical-speak at dinners. The Greenman family's commitment to their family, friends, and patients has long been an example for me. My parents, Paula and Achille, my grandparents, and my brothers, Owen and Patrick, taught me not to sit still when you see wrong. They showed, through their examples, how to make your vocations and avocations bring forth love and justice in the world. My daughter, Madeleine, fills me with hope for the future. And Paul Farmer, my late mentor and so much of my inspiration to become a doctor, taught me to fear no one, to make a preferential option for the poor, and to always work alongside friends.

Introduction

The usual forms having been gone through, the body of Samuel Pickwick was soon afterwards confided to the custody of the tipstaff, to be by him taken to the warden of the Fleet Prison, and there detained until the amount of the damages and costs in the action of Bardell against Pickwick was fully paid and satisfied. "And that," said Mr. Pickwick, laughing, "will be a very long time."
— Charles Dickens, *The Pickwick Papers*

The ultimate, hidden truth of the world is that it is something that we make, and could just as easily make differently.
— David Graeber, *The Utopia of Rules*

In the laundry of the Danville Regional Medical Center in southern Virginia in 1995, Ms. Wilson folded hospital gowns. Five days a week, it was her task to turn the piles of dirty laundry, towels, gowns, and scrubs into neat, clean stacks. At age 68, she was older than most people who performed such relentless physical labor. She had not planned to have such a job at her age. And, to be honest, it was not a job, not really, for at the end of each week, the hospital did not send her a paycheck.

Grieving the recent death of her husband after a prolonged hospitalization, Ms. Wilson faced medical debt she could never hope to repay on her fixed income. Danville gave her the option of entering its "Service-Credit Program," in which patients owing between $300 and $20,000 were put to work typing, filing, housekeeping, landscaping, and printing. For their labor, they earned $5 per hour toward settling their debts. "Net pay is applied directly to the bill, so no cash changes hands," explained an upbeat front-page article in the *Richmond Times-Dispatch*.[1] Nowhere in the article was the possibility mentioned that the medical center, a nonprofit, could simply write off the unpaid debts of low-income patients as charity-care. Later in the article, the Service-Credit Program was lauded as a "working cure," without a hint of irony.

Perhaps most striking was the fact that the hospital leadership was proud of this program. It was, after all, a rather dystopian scheme that would recoup, through the manual labor of a poor widow, the costs incurred during the medical care of her late husband. It helped low-income patients "who want to retain their dignity and protect their credit rating and do the right thing about eliminating a bill," said one hospital executive. He bragged that they had fielded inquiries from 40 hospitals about starting similar initiatives. Dr. Thomas Massaro, a pediatrician and health policy scholar at the University of Virginia, called the Service-Credit Program "ingenious" for the "mindset it establishes in the patient population, that there are ways of exercising responsibility and control over your destiny."[2]

How could such a program come to be seen as a benefit to patients? In what kind of society would this modern-day indentured servitude win laudatory publicity from the regional newspaper and plaudits from health policy experts? To really see how this is possible, you have to understand what alternatives indebted patients faced, what repercussions they could expect if they did not take hospitals such as Danville up on their offers of unpaid labor. Facing an impending future of ruined credit, harassing phone calls, and legal trouble, Ms. Wilson decided that working in the hospital laundry, inhumane and unremunerated as it was, was the best among her very bad options.

There has always been inhumanity in American medical care. Society's marginalized have long dealt with varied forms of neglect and exploitation. But beginning in the 1980s, a rise in unpaid medical bills occurred alongside a transformation in how hospitals, including nonprofit hospitals, try to collect those debts. This book tells the story of how the collection of medical debt in the United States came to be so aggressive, and of the impact this is having on Americans' lives. For centuries, doctors were often unable to collect—or declined to pursue—unpaid bills. But during the past four decades, such debts in America have shifted from obligations negotiated by doctors and patients and hospitals into assets bought and sold by people with no role at all in patient care. Spurred in part by insurance companies' turn toward higher co-payments and deductibles, hospitals faced more severely delinquent payments. Hospital administrators turned away from charity-care and gave in to the siren call of collection companies, including debt buyers and collection attorneys.

Whereas for most of the twentieth century much of the work of collecting delinquent payments was done by hospitals' own in-house collection departments, by the early twenty-first century many hospitals had come to rely on outside agencies and debt buyers. Here is how the system works: Hospitals "assign" their debts to a collection agency; the agency works the debt and keeps a portion of what they successfully recoup. Sometimes hospitals sell their debt, in which case they receive an up-front payment and the buyer keeps all of the money collected thereafter. How common are these arrangements? As early as 2013, hospitals and health care providers were the largest group of customers for collection agencies and agencies' largest source of recoveries in dollar terms.[3] By 2018, a survey of 100 hospital executives found that 54 percent used a third-party vendor for at least a portion of their debt collection.[4] In 2020 alone, medical debt collection brought in $1.5 billion in revenue for America's 7,000 debt collection agencies.[5]

Hospitals and debt collectors have a variety of tactics to get patients to pay up. The simplest and oldest methods involved chastising letters, home visits, and phone calls. If this was not enough, they reported the delinquent debt to credit bureaus. But when this proved ineffective, as it often did for debts that the patient simply could not pay, collectors turned to increasingly aggressive tactics. They filed lawsuits against patients and then sought to enforce payment. They did this by claiming a portion of patients' paychecks (wage garnishment), by emptying their bank accounts (bank executions), or even by kicking them out of their homes (property foreclosure). If patients did not appear in court, collectors sometimes asked judges to arrest the patients and put them in jail (body attachment). These actions, in addition to selling debt, reporting to credit bureaus, and refusing to provide care until debts are paid, are known as "extraordinary collection actions," and they have become all too ordinary. Between 2018 and 2020, 26 of the 100 largest hospitals in the United States filed lawsuits to collect bills owed by their patients.[6] Among a representative sample of hospitals surveyed in 2021 and 2022, more than two-thirds had policies that included taking legal actions such as lawsuits, wage garnishment, and property liens against patients in debt.[7]

The debt collection industry is one of the many intermediaries in health care, alongside private equity, insurance companies, and pharmacy benefit managers, that profit off sickness while doing little to treat it. Bringing debt collectors into the billing relationship between doctors and patients was not a benign exercise. Divorced from any clinical or social bonds to patients, collectors of debt used draconian tactics. These became the norm, and hospitals, too, abandoned lenience. Hospitals and their collectors reported patients to credit bureaus, harming their chances for home mortgages and jobs. They sued patients, adding legal woes to physical illness. After winning these cases, as they almost always did, hospitals and their agents garnished patients' wages, seized their bank accounts, and even foreclosed on their homes. In extreme cases, police showed up at the homes of patients who did not appear in court for these cases in order to bring them to jail. Hospitals used the might of the state to discipline the patient in debt. Those unfortunate enough to face destitution and illness at the same time were, in effect, treated like criminals.

Even when hospitals had charity-care programs in place, many qualifying patients were pursued for these debts, often because they had not been informed about financial assistance or did not have the wherewithal to complete the application. This unmerciful attitude to debtor patients conflicted with the reigning vision of nonprofit hospitals as pillars of community service and charity. In a rational response to the cascade of misery that could follow unpaid bills, low-income patients delayed necessary care. Their wounds festered; their cancers metastasized.

Press coverage of debt collection tactics proved a public relations debacle for hospitals. In the mid-2000s and again in the late 2010s, the burden of debt on patients became the focus of investigative journalists at local and national publications. In these moments, legislators and regulators at the state and federal levels launched investigations and proposed new laws. In response, administrators began to publicize other, more "dignified" means of debt repayment, such as making widows work in the laundry room. The modern hospital emerged from the medieval almshouse, but today it can resemble another relic—the debtor prison.

Various state and federal regulations and laws have tinkered at the edges of this problem: forbidding collectors from verbally abusing patients over the phone, requiring hospitals to have written charity-care policies, and, more recently, limiting reporting of medical debt to credit bureaus. But consumer protections in the legal code aim mostly to encourage collectors to maintain a certain decorum over the phone. Here is an example: The Fair Debt Collection Practices Act of 1977, the major legislative protection for consumers, allows debt collectors to threaten to take a patient to court, but only if the threat is real. The real roots of the problem, the onerous debts and the aggressive tactics to collect, have continued.

I am an emergency doctor and a historian. I have seen the impact of debt collection on my patients; in fact, I feared losing my job when I spoke up about lawsuits against patients filed by my own hospital's collection agency. I wrote this book to explain something I am witnessing firsthand—in the United States, debt and debt collection are changing the most important relationships in medicine, driving a wedge between doctors and patients by destroying patients' trust that medical professionals are looking out for their best interests. Worse, debt collection ruins patients' financial lives, and the fear of this ruination keeps many from seeking care when they need it.

This is a story that has been told in pieces. It appears in outrageous stories in major newspapers, in stump speeches by Bernie Sanders and Elizabeth Warren, in congressional hearings, and in television segments on John Oliver's *Last Week Tonight*. The *New York Times*, ProPublica, *Kaiser Health News*, NPR, the *Washington Post*, and the *Wall Street Journal*, and many other media organizations have written about hospitals that sue patients, seek to shirk charity-care obligations, and charge outrageously high bills to low-income patients. Videos about medical debt and how to deal with collectors have been seen by millions of people on social media platforms such as TikTok and YouTube. Medical debt has recently gained sustained attention in medical and public health journals, with studies of the extent of debt and of the collection tactics taken by hospitals. Organized efforts have been launched to forgive debts through charitable efforts such as RIP Medical Debt or to challenge the very legitimacy of medical debt through groups such as the Debt Collective, an outgrowth of the Occupy Wall Street movement.

But the story of medical debt and its collection has yet to be told all at once, in a way that explains how medical debt became so gargantuan, and how an industry developed to collect it. This history encompasses law, finance, and medicine. It is a tale of swashbuckling entrepreneurship, of ruthless empire-building, of infuriating bureaucracy, and of dogged protest. But most surprising of all, it is a story about blindness. Even as the amount of medical debt came to reach hundreds of billions of dollars, and as local hospitals sued patients by the thousands, most doctors and even administrators knew little about what their patients were facing.

In the meantime, medical debt has become a behemoth. Tallies vary, depending on whether you count medical debt placed on credit cards, or borrowed from friends, or in payment plans, or all bills past due, or just those delinquent debts that are reported to credit bureaus, but a 2022 survey estimated that 100 million Americans carry medical debt in some form.[8] A 2021 study with a more restricted definition, including only medical debt in collections that appeared on Americans' credit reports, totaled $140 billion. This study found that 17.8 percent of Americans had medical debt in collections. The average person owed $429 of medical debt, more than every other source of debt combined ($390).[9] Other experts on medical debt, including Senator Elizabeth Warren, have encouraged an even more expansive definition, arguing that lost income due to illness and caregiving responsibilities places even greater burdens on American families than direct charges from health care.[10]

Debt is a scary subject, one so many of us live with but try not to think too much about. It fills us with a deep sense of dread, of foreboding, of the sense that our lives and our freedom are being sapped. We have been led to think of it as something that we, as individuals, bring upon ourselves. Our inability to repay debts fills us with guilt; that guilt is a potent force for collectors, who insist that their work confers dignity on delinquent debtors. But when people are brought to court or lose their homes over hospital bills, how much dignity can they really have? As the anthropologist David Graeber observed in a magisterial global history of debt,

> If history shows anything, it is that there's no better way to justify relations founded on violence, to make such relations seem moral, than by reframing them in the language of debt—above all, because it immediately makes it seem that it's the victim who's doing something wrong.[11]

While personal irresponsibility is nowhere near a sufficient explanation for the rising burden of consumer debt, it explains next to nothing when it comes to medical debt. These debts are almost entirely outside of an individual's control and fall most heavily on the most vulnerable. Medical debt and aggressive collection are widespread, but they are not a universal experience. Like other hardships in American life, their frequency rises as one moves further down the steep gradient of historically determined inequality. In March 2022, the Consumer Financial Protection Bureau (CFPB) reported that 43 million Americans had medical debt on their credit reports. These debts were particularly prevalent among Black (28 percent) and Hispanic (22 percent) Americans, whereas White (17 percent) Americans experienced such debt less frequently.[12] Other studies have found additional factors that render people more likely to be in medical debt, including living with a disability,[13] living in a low-income zip code,[14] living in a state that did not expand Medicaid after the passage of the Affordable Care Act,[15] and being a woman.[16] Many of these disparities are long-standing; studies in the 1980s and 1990s found that pregnancy and childbirth were the most common diagnoses for patients who ended up with unpaid bills.[17] Regional variations in medical debt are massive, with much higher burdens in the South. Among the 20 most populous counties in the United States, the percentage of people reporting medical debt ranged from a low of 3 percent of respondents in New York County, home of Manhattan, to a high of 27.3 percent in Tarrant County, Texas, home of Fort Worth.[18]

This book has surprisingly few bona fide individual villains. There are some very wealthy debt collectors whose actions do seem to fit into any reasonable definition of greed, but they are relatively small in number. The rank-and-file debt collectors who make the phone calls that so many of us dread are generally working-class Americans who struggle with their own debts. There are hospital administrators who do seem strangely enthusiastic about using exploitative tactics to collect from vulnerable patients, but most sincerely believe they are trying to be fiscally responsible when they hound patients to pay unaffordable debts.

But let us agree, from the start, that they are misguided. First, not all hospitals are in financial trouble. In 2019, America's hospitals recorded their highest average profit margin ever, at 6.7 percent. And while many hospitals struggled during the early days of the COVID-19 pandemic, massive federal support led them to finish 2020 with similar profit margins as they had in 2019.[19]

Of course, there are many hospitals that do not operate with such comfortable margins. Some struggle to stay afloat, and every year there are closures, depriving local residents of a life-saving resource and an important source of employment. But pursuing patients who cannot afford to pay does precious little to help. TransUnion Healthcare reports that in 2016, 68 percent of hospital bills under $500 were not paid in full. Heftier bills were even less likely to be paid, with 99 percent of hospital bills over $3,000 not paid in full.[20] Other estimates are even more dismal: Crystal Ewing, manager of data integrity at a billing software firm called Zirmed, estimates that uninsured patients pay only 6 percent of what they are billed.[21] This meager repayment is the reason hospitals will accept mere cents on the dollar when they sell their debt to outside buyers. It makes sense that uninsured and underinsured patients are not able to afford out-of-pocket bills; roughly half of Americans say they have difficulty finding the money to pay for a $400 emergency expense. Most patients in arrears just do not have the money to pay without risking their financial health, a truth that has given rise to an adage long in use among hospital administrators: "Self-pay equals no pay."[22]

Suing patients does not meaningfully contribute to a hospital's financial well-being. A 2017 study of Virginia hospitals that garnished the wages of patients found that they collected, on average, 0.1 percent of hospital revenue through this practice.[23] Even the hospital that sued the most patients in the state, Mary Washington Hospital in Fredericksburg, gained only 0.2 percent of its revenue from wage garnishments.[24] Marty Makary, the senior author on the study, pointed out that on average, hospitals that sued patients collected less than health system chief executive officers typically earn in a year. "The argument that we have to do something this ugly in order to stay afloat is not supported by the data," he said.[25] For the struggling hospital, suing low-income patients is akin to using a bucket to bail water out of a sinking cruise ship, and then throwing the water into a crowded lifeboat. And most often it is not the financially insecure safety-net or rural access hospital filling the court dockets. Institutions that pursue patients aggressively frequently have comfortable operating margins and well-paid executives.[26]

Beyond the fact that they do not solve a hospital's financial problems, there are three additional major problems with aggressive medical debt collection.

The first is that medical debt does tremendous harm to patients' financial well-being. Perhaps the easiest way to see how much damage has been done to those who owe medical debt is to see what it has cost them. A 2019 survey found that 16 percent of Americans had put off major household purchases to pay medical bills, while 12 percent had used up most of their savings and 9 percent had increased their credit card debt.[27] Americans with new medical debt are at increased risk of food insecurity, eviction, and foreclosure.[28] A 2018 survey found that most respondents feared the costs associated with a serious illness more than a serious illness itself.[29] The burdens of medical debt fall hardest on people who are already in arrears; according to an analysis of 2018 Census Bureau survey data, 79 percent of medical debt is held by people with zero or negative net worth.[30]

The second problem is that medical debt prevents patients from accessing necessary medical care. Hospitals are allowed to refuse to care for patients with outstanding debts, as long as the patients do not have an emergency. But even if they are not refused care outright, patients in arrears will avoid an encounter that only further increases their shame and debt.[31] We have known this for some time, and we keep relearning it. The RAND Health Insurance Experiment, conducted in the 1970s, found that low-income Americans with high blood pressure experienced a 10 percent increase in the likelihood of death if they were enrolled in health insurance plans with high out-of-pocket payments.[32] In 2005, a survey found that non-elderly Americans who reported problems with medical bills were more than six times as likely to have skipped a medical test, treatment, or follow-up.[33] Another study published in 2013 found that compared to respondents with no medical debt, those with medical debt had 3.3 times greater odds of forgoing care.[34] A rigorous econometric analysis of a financial assistance program in Northern California published in 2021 found that low-income people who qualified for debt relief and elimination of cost-sharing were far more likely to seek medical care than patients with slightly higher incomes, who did not qualify for the financial assistance. This difference had profound consequences: The slightly lower-income patients who qualified for financial assistance were, the researchers found, benefiting from diagnosis and management of treatable conditions.[35]

The third problem with medical debt is that it destroys the trust that makes medical care both morally meaningful and physiologically effective. How likely are you to listen to a doctor when you suspect their recommendation, if followed, will land you in a courtroom or cause you to lose your home? Will you really believe your best interest is their main concern? Even if you trust your doctor, will you believe the hospital is looking out for patients, rather than its own bottom line? Speaking of hospitals, Georgia State University law professor Erin Fuse Brown argued that "there has to be a balance between getting their bills paid but also being a reasonable community member."[36]

The public has already lost trust in hospital leadership. Whereas 70 percent of respondents in a nationwide survey conducted in 2021 reported trusting physicians "to do what is right for you and your family" at least "most of the time," only 22 percent professed such trust in hospital executives.[37] Administrators do not generally inspire the same confidence as caring professionals, but this is a striking disparity, and one that may eventually drag down trust in doctors and nurses, particularly as more clinicians come under the control of corporate entities such as mammoth hospital systems and private equity companies.

In this book, I am most interested in answering the following questions: How did it come to pass that so many patients are being pursued so aggressively for medical debts? Who is involved in this debt collection? And what does it do to patients and to the people who work in medicine? Why would hospitals, and particularly private nonprofit hospitals, which are associated in the public imagination with community solidarity, with care without regard to means to pay, of philanthropy and fellow feeling, resort to aggressive collection tactics? Why would their leaders sell patients' debts, or take patients to court, or seize their bank accounts and wages and homes, or throw them in jail, particularly when hospitals gain little revenue from these tactics? And why would the medical professionals who work at these institutions permit the ruin of their most vulnerable patients?

This history will focus in large part on private nonprofit hospitals. Why this focus, when outpatient physicians' offices also sometimes resort to lawsuits, and for-profit hospitals have been aggressive collectors? First, nonprofit hospitals are the backbone of acute care in the United States. In 2022, whereas 18.5 percent of community hospitals (a term that excludes federal government hospitals and psychiatric hospitals) were owned by state or local governments and 23.9 percent were for-profit, 57.6 percent were private nonprofit hospitals.[38] Historically known as "voluntary" or charity hospitals, the private nonprofits are the places that Americans most often turn to in times of unexpected severe illness, when they are at their most vulnerable. Unlike pharmaceutical companies or even private doctors' offices, they have forsworn profits. They have no shareholders demanding payouts. Instead, they find their historical origins in almshouses, ethnic community associations, and religious institutions. They are exempt from taxation specifically because of the community benefits they promise to provide. In a capitalist society driven by the profit motive, nonprofit hospitals profess to stand apart, to be driven not by private avarice but by communal care. They are also the institutions that train the majority of America's physicians, and for certain specialties, including mine (emergency medicine), they are where most doctors are employed. In addition, hospitalization accounts for a disproportionate share of catastrophic medical expenditures, the types that are hardest to repay and most likely to result in aggressive collections.[39]

This is not an easy history to study. Discerning how much different patients with various health insurance plans, or none, were made to pay for medical care is no simple task, particularly given the unique list prices used by each hospital and discounts negotiated by each insurer. Likewise, tallying all the debts from medical costs, as well as lost earnings due to illness and caregiving responsibilities, can be challenging. Consumers without sufficient savings often try to pay medical bills with credit cards, payday loans, or, if they are lucky, loans from family or friends, none of which are easy data to disentangle.

There is a record trail that details the impact of medical debt on individual lives, but it is not complete. Federal bankruptcy court records list payments owed by filers to medical supply companies, private physicians, and hospitals. But these records are not saved permanently. The records of small claims courts detail the lawsuits hospitals file against patients for payment, as well as hospitals' responses to patients' pleas for leniency, but these records are not fully digitized. Debt collectors and hospital administrators are not the most willing interview subjects. They have come to fear media coverage, which can bring unwelcome scrutiny by regulators and frighten potential clients. I did speak with industry veterans, but many were well-versed in public relations and were not inclined to answer my questions directly. Mostly they turned to talking points, about good intentions as well as the supposed benefits of debt collection for health care providers in particular and the economy in general.

The very lexicon of the industry is full of euphemism and obfuscation. After critical press attention, the Debt Buyers Association renamed itself the Receivables Management Association. Practitioners of billing and collections now refer to their work as "revenue cycle management." As George Orwell explained, "such phraseology is needed if one wants to name things without calling up mental pictures of them."[40]

So to tell the story of medical debt collection, I had to look beyond these sources. Some of the most useful were trade journals produced by associations of health care executives and debt collectors. In these industry periodicals, professionals wrote with candor about challenges and plans. Other sources included court records from hospital lawsuits, collection companies' earnings calls with investors, local newspapers, congressional testimony, and my own participant observation as an emergency physician.

This is not a book about every facet or pathology of American health care. The pricing of pharmaceuticals, the tactics of insurance companies to maximize profits, the political power of medical specialty societies, and the way care is unequally distributed and utilized are discussed, but mainly as they relate to the central issues of this book: the rise of medical debts owed by patients to hospitals and doctors, the tactics used to collect that debt, and the effect that this problem has on patients. Some parts of the health care system are so inextricably linked to this problem that they have to be discussed in some detail. For instance, changes in federal and state funding for hospital care beginning in the 1980s left hospitals with more unreimbursed expenses. As a result, hospitals pursued patients more aggressively for repayment. The increasing problem of uninsurance in the United States during the 1980s and 1990s contributed to medical debt, while the incomplete Medicaid expansion after the Affordable Care Act led to vast geographic disparities in medical debt among low-income Americans.

A number of broader social forces have contributed to this transformation of medical debt. These include structural racism, economic inequality, the late-twentieth-century rise of neoliberal ideology, early twenty-first century efforts to organize health care workers, social movements such as Occupy Wall Street, and shifts in health financing and ownership. There are many causes of medical debt's growing role in Americans' lives. This book is not a minute analysis of every law and regulation related to the rise of medical debt, but I do focus on shifts in third-party financing, health insurance reimbursement, social insurance, financialization, and privatization that have propelled medical debt ever upwards. These are all essential parts of the story; the rise of medical debt markets in the United States, and their disproportionate impact on the disenfranchised, can scarcely be understood without discussing them.

But for an issue as (seemingly) abstruse and complex as secondary markets for medical debt, there is value in the immediacy of human stories. Who are the debt collectors? What are they like? What do they want? Beyond the aggregate statistics that appear in headlines, how does debt affect actual, flesh-and-blood people? Aggressive medical debt collection has impoverished many, caused people to have their wages and bank accounts and homes confiscated, and kept some from the life-saving care they might otherwise have received. There are enormous human stakes in the structural, historical, and legal analyses in this book. This is not a dry, simple, or straightforward story. It is heartbreaking and infuriating.

Nor is this a how-to guide for those suffering from medical debt. Those do exist, and some of the people involved in creating those guides are part of this narrative.[41] My hope is that this book will deepen our understanding of where this problem came from so that we can help people struggling with medical debt, preferably by doing away with it altogether. This sounds grandiose, I am sure. There are already people working to make this a reality, but we will need more, many more.

There is always a risk that a story like this will read as a morality tale rather than a balanced account of the rise of aggressive medical debt collection and the environment in which this was allowed to occur. I admit to a point of view on this topic, one influenced by my own sense of morality and my experiences as a physician. As I recount later, poor patients at my own hospital were pursued in court for medical debt. When I went public with my concerns, hospital administrators insisted I was out of line. But I certainly do not intend to portray all physicians as valiant and all hospital administrators as villainous. This would be both wrong and unhelpful.

Most of the actors in this story were simply doing their jobs, as they understood them. Hospital financial administrators and staff, especially at nonprofit hospitals, have had reason to worry about uncollectible debts and rising costs, and many are trying mightily to keep their doors open. Doctors, for their part, have had precious little to say about this problem. Few inquire about the billing practices of their hospitals, and those who do know what is going on risk antagonizing their employers, and losing their jobs, if they speak up. We all find ways to rationalize our everyday actions and inactions. Uncovering these justifications is also a part of the story.

I am not an impartial observer, but I did strive to ensure that the perspectives and concerns of diverse actors were fairly represented. I interviewed everyone I could, and gave all of the significant characters in the book a chance to tell their stories for themselves. Some would not answer my calls and emails. In those cases, as in everything I wrote, I worked to ensure that all claims were backed by credible sources.

The physician–patient relationship is a particular concern of mine, impelled in large part by my interactions with patients concerned about the effects of my care on their families' financial well-being. This is an important part of the story, as financialization has made a tradable commodity of obligations that were once intensely personal relationships built on trust. This has unique consequences for health care, a sphere no one can avoid and one in which almost every patient is in a position of vulnerability. This more impersonal age of health financing, in which responsibility for dealing with patient-debtors has been handed over to collectors whose sole imperative is to secure as much money as possible, has been a powerful force in the metastasizing damage done by medical debts.

The book is organized into three main parts. The first chronicles the development of our system of debt collection up until the dawn of the twenty-first century. Chapter 1 shows how during much of the nineteenth and early twentieth centuries, doctors struggled to organize an even remotely standardized billing system and insisted—although they often did not live up to the pledge—that the poor should be given free or discounted care. Over time, however, the cost of new technologies increased, threatening patients with financial ruin even after their ills were cured. Private and public insurance schemes were devised to protect against these disasters, but unlike most other industrialized countries of this period, the United States never guaranteed universal coverage, and medical debt drove people to desperate acts.

Next, in Chapter 2, I come to the 1980s and 1990s, when a slowdown in federal and state support for the care of the poor and decreasing reimbursements for the privately insured led to an increase in uncompensated care costs for American hospitals. To recoup some of their debts, hospitals and doctors' offices turned patients away at their doors and relied increasingly on collections agencies. Medical debt was fast becoming a significant part of the portfolios of debt collectors, whose phone calls and letters and visits became a recurring feature of the lives of poor patients. By the 1990s, this debt began to be bundled and sold on private financial markets.

The second part of the book tells the stories of some of the major figures in medical debt collection at the start of the twenty-first century, including debt collectors and debt buyers, prominent hospital systems that turned to aggressive collection tactics, the journalists who uncovered these tactics and their effects on patients, and the activists who fought to protect patients. Chapter 3 chronicles the rise of the medical debt collection industry by profiling a few of its titans, including a rags-to-riches empire builder, a National Basketball Association team owner, and a disgraced member of Congress. Divorced from any clinical or social bonds to patients, collectors and purchasers of debt could be particularly aggressive, using harassing phone calls, credit reports, and legal action to secure payment of debts. This chapter shows the fortunes to be made from debt collection and the consequences for real people when patients become prey.

Eventually, the pursuit of patients for unpaid bills drew too much outrage to be ignored. Chapter 4 follows the effects of public advocacy and a series of exposés by the *Wall Street Journal* in 2003, focused in large part on the aggressive debt collection practices of Yale University's major teaching hospital. In the months after these articles, a congressional committee held a series of hearings in which a Republican chairman sought to shame doctors and hospitals into being less punitive about debt collection. He highlighted wild particularities of medical debt, such as the practice of pursuing people for the debts of their spouses.

Have we made any progress? The third part of the book discusses what has changed, for better and for worse, in the years since the passage of the Affordable Care Act in 2010, as well as the range of ideas from reform to radical change. Chapter 5 explains how the Affordable Care Act and the CFPB tried to remedy some of the major problems with medical debt by expanding health insurance coverage and by mandating closer enforcement of charity-care rules; nevertheless, aggressive debt collection tactics endured. As with many pathologies of American life, the pain of medical debt followed the fault lines of class, race, and gender.

Chapter 6 highlights some of the people working to change the system, including former debt collectors and hospital administrators who have used their knowledge to press for reform, a former bartender who seeks to get patients out from under mountains of debt, nursing unions organizing to stop aggressive debt collection, and activists seeking to abolish medical debt altogether.

In the Conclusion, I discuss the perils of cynicism and the possibility of an America without medical debt. Finally, in the Afterword, I turn toward the personal. As a resident in emergency medicine training in Rhode Island in 2019, I was surprised, and horrified, to learn that my care might put patients in legal trouble. Like most of my colleagues, I assumed our nonprofit teaching hospitals forgave the debts of patients who could not pay their bills. When I found out that my hospital system sued poor patients and garnished their wages, I wrote a critical piece on a local blog. Thus began a series of acrimonious exchanges with the hospital leadership who, after accusing me of spreading falsehoods, eventually halted its practice.

Although I want everyone to read this book, I really do hope that health care workers will find something particularly useful in it. Doctors, nurses, and other professionals involved in direct care of patients generally have little to do with billing and collections. We almost never know how much patients will be charged for the care they receive, nor do we know about the work of our billing departments.[42] Most of us know about the Emergency Medical Treatment and Active Labor Act, the federal law stating that hospitals with emergency departments must provide a medical screening exam to any patient and, if an emergency condition exists, must stabilize the patient or transfer them to another facility, regardless of ability to pay. Most of us are vaguely aware that charity-care exists for the poorest patients, although for the most part we are not able to tell our patients who qualifies or how to obtain it.

Yet we cannot claim perpetual ignorance; that time has come and gone. Aggressive medical debt collection does not keep hospital doors open, and it certainly does not pad our salaries, but it does do violence to our patients and undoes the work of healing that health care workers struggle so hard at each day. By burdening patients with psychological stress and financial harm, by frightening them away from care they need, by destroying their trust in medical institutions, and by seizing their wages, their savings, their shelter, and even their freedom, medical debt collection works against our patients' well-being. It attacks what is best in the profession of medicine: the idea that the patients' interests ultimately supersede all else.

PART I

The Backstory: Collecting Medical Debt in Nineteenth- and Twentieth-Century America

CHAPTER 1
Before the Debt Machine

It requires no scientific training, no love for humanity, no toil, no self-sacrifice, to buy up the necessities of life while they are cheap, operate and combine with others to put up the price to the highest possible limit, and then sell out. . . . And yet society affords these men every luxury and extravagance . . . while it sends the indispensable doctor forth on his life-saving, Heaven-ordained errand of mercy and usefulness at all hours of the day and night, during all seasons of the year and in all kinds of weather, and yet begrudges him the modicum necessary to keep himself and his family in respectable comfort.
  —John J. Taylor, MD, *The Physician as a Business Man*

Every nineteenth-century novel you crack open may delude you at first with tales of love and romance, but at the core of each one lies a bank account. Or the lack of one.
  —Margaret Atwood, *Payback: Debt and the Shadow Side of Wealth*

Everyone will tell you that that time before the time you are at any given place is the best.
  —Isaac Fitzgerald, *Dirtbag, Massachusetts: A Confessional*

Today's medical debt collection complex is a recent invention. Before the mid-twentieth century, medical billing in the United States often intensely personal and morally fraught negotiations between doctors and patients. Meanwhile, state laws across the country, inspired by opposition to old English debtors' prisons, prohibited aggressive debt collection measures such as wage garnishment. But as medicine became more organized, centralized, and expensive, medical debt became a growing problem in Americans' lives.

Medical debts often proved difficult to collect for many of the same reasons as other kinds of debt. Many colonial settlers were Old World debtors who had fled the specter of debtors' prisons. As a result, bankruptcy laws set forth in the colonies were slightly more forgiving to debtors than in England.[1] They were, on the other hand, unforgiving toward physicians thought to be fleecing their patients. A Virginia law passed in 1646 even allowed for the arrest of any physician or surgeon who charged "immoderate and excessive rates."[2]

Debt remained at the forefront of the political agenda during the early years of the young nation. In 1786, after local courts in western Massachusetts ruled to foreclose on farmers' land, popular unrest spread in the region. Local militias refused to move against the rebels. The debtors, many of whom were Revolutionary War veterans who had returned home owed back pay and owing onerous new taxes, garnered the sympathies of locally influential figures. Dr. William Whiting, a doctor who also served as Chief Justice of Berkshire County, wrote in their defense, denouncing the creditor elite as a class of "overgrown plunderers."[3] Bostonian aristocrats called for troops from other states to put down what became known as "Shays Rebellion," named after Daniel Shays, a farmer and Revolutionary soldier who helped lead the revolt. The revolt was eventually put down, but it so frightened George Washington and other founders that it helped spur the abandonment of the Articles of Confederation in favor of a stronger federal Constitution.

Although by modern standards laws against debtors were harsh, the trend toward more rights for debtors continued during the nineteenth century. The first bankruptcy statute after Independence, signed into law by John Adams in 1800, allowed debtors to initiate bankruptcy proceedings and discharge their debts. Policies were more liberal on the American frontier, where settlers journeyed in search of relief during periods of economic depression. In the aftermath of the Panic of 1819, for instance, Kentucky, Tennessee, Missouri, and Illinois passed relief measures such as "stay laws" that allowed debtors time before creditors could enforce collections and seize property.[4]

The laws of what was known then as the American West soon influenced federal statutes. The state of Kentucky outlawed debtors' prisons in 1821.[5] When Andrew Jackson of Tennessee ran for presidency later that decade, he railed against the practice of jailing debtors.[6] In his 1831 State of the Union Address, he declared, "The personal liberty of the citizen seems too sacred to be held, as in many cases it now is, at the will of the creditor."[7] In 1833, the US Congress outlawed debtors' prisons, 4 years before Charles Dickens scandalized the British public with his depiction of one in his first novel, *The Pickwick Papers*.[8]

Creditors in America may not have been as powerful as they had been across the Atlantic, yet they were not impotent. They could sue debtors or turn to other degrading tactics. Some would hire a "bawler-out," usually a woman with a loud voice and a penchant for witty insults, to stand outside the debtor's home or workplace and decry him, his friends, and his family for his delinquency.[9] Still, empty threats could only go so far. As historian Tamara Plakins Thornton details in a history of farm loans in the first half of the nineteenth century, large companies attempted to ensure punctual repayment by sending notices threatening lawsuits, but rarely followed through for fear of popular opposition to actual foreclosures.[10]

Physicians also found themselves among this class of frustrated creditors. In the medical journals of the nineteenth century, private practice physicians complained they could not earn a decent living because patients did not pay promptly for their care. An 1825 editorial in *The New England Journal of Medicine and Surgery* lamented, "It is in no degree the custom to settle professional accounts at any particular period. The common practice is to let them alone, and suffer them to accumulate indefinitely." Physicians, the editorial continued, often died in debt, having received from patients only some small portion of their bills, often through payments in kind rather than cash. "Now this is not well," the editors complained. "It diminishes the wider influence which [the physician], as a man of learning and of reputation, should exert about him."[11]

Beginning in the eighteenth century and with increasing frequency during the first decades of the nineteenth century, medical societies formed in cities and states across the country, often with the major aim of enforcing standardized fee schedules among their members. In New York City, Philadelphia, Washington, DC, Boston, and Vermont, among many other places, physicians sought to establish a fee-for-service system, in which payments were made at the point of care or at regular intervals.[12] The societies hoped this would replace "contracts for annual attendance," in which individuals or families paid a predetermined fee for all necessary care from their physician each year.

But in some major cities where they undertook these efforts, doctors faced a problem of oversupply. They struggled to enforce higher and more uniform fees during a period when the medical marketplace was fiercely competitive, because the number of practitioners was high relative to the number of people who could afford their attention. As a result, the new fee schedules were aspirational rather than reality. In the words of one Boston physician, they were "stuff that dreams are made of, the basis for air-castles, *châteaux en Espagne*."[13]

Even as they tried to increase physician incomes, medical societies acknowledged the need to provide care regardless of ability to pay. Philadelphia's College of Physicians' *Rules for Professional Conduct*, published in 1843, advised the following:

> The poor . . . ought to be deemed the objects of kindness and attention; and to them gratuitous services should be rendered with promptness and alacrity. In the consideration of fees, let it be remembered, that although mean ones from the affluent are bust and degrading, yet the characteristical beneficence of the profession is inconsistent with sordid views, and avaricious rapacity.[14]

Cincinnati's 1859 fee schedule made another solemn promise to treat the indigent: "We will . . . (as we have ever done), exercise clemency toward those less favored by Providence and will give our time and strength willingly and cheerfully to the suffering poor, without a wish for compensation."[15] Doctors sought to assure the public that their professional responsibilities included free care for the poor.

When physicians could not collect from patients they deemed able to pay, they sometimes turned to county officers or independent arbitrators to enforce debt repayment. However, as Dr. George Wilson of Port Huron, Michigan, complained in 1862, in these settings they found little to defend themselves against patients' frequent claims that their fees were exorbitant.[16] So exasperated was one physician with his inability to collect that he took to anonymously publishing his lament in verse in the *St. Louis Medical and Surgical Journal*:

> Book, oh doctor! Book your fee!
> Charge—I'll pay it futurely,
> When the crops all by are laid,
> When every other bill is paid,
> (Or when of death again afraid)
> I'll pay it—grudgingly.[17]

In 1892, Philadelphia physician John Jay Taylor published a manual for his fellow doctors who had trouble collecting. He instructed them to be more diligent and less forgiving with their billing. He recommended they send monthly bills and refuse to treat "systematic deadbeats." He proposed a scheme of "mutual protection," wherein doctors would combine to form a "collections committee" tasked with sending letters to "delinquents."[18] Patients in arrears who were deemed able to pay would be required to settle accounts before receiving care from any physician.

Doctors should, Taylor allowed, provide some charity-care, but they should avoid too much lenience for those who claimed to be "hard up." These patients were "waiting for the easy time, and this time comes to but few."[19] Because almost everyone was struggling financially, the doctor had to be firm even with those who claimed to be down on their luck.

Taylor complained that the law made it too difficult to collect. He was particularly agitated by the fact that patients threatened with wage garnishment or property seizure were legally allowed to claim exemptions, allowing them to keep some of their property and wages. Physicians' bills, he argued, should be excepted from these laws, allowing doctors to seize otherwise exempted property.

Unlike private physician practices, hospitals were initially focused on the care of the poor, and they did not rely on paying patients to keep their doors open. Urban hospitals in the nineteenth-century United States were funded mainly by donations and built with large open wards to be filled with charity patients. But application had to be made for admission, and only those deemed sufficiently blameless and industrious would be allowed in. Patients might be turned away for perceived drunkenness, mental illness, or any other form of unworthiness. Rhode Island Hospital, built after the Civil War with donations from the state's wealthy industrialists, had such a policy. In 1872, Robert Hale Ives, the hospital's first president and a partner at his family shipping, textile, and banking business Brown & Ives, described the motivations for the hospital's policy of discrimination:

> It is not an asylum for the poor, nor a receptacle for incurables; still less is it a refuge for the vicious, the fallen and the degraded. Much as this class of persons are to be pitied, and much as they need aid, this Hospital is not the place for them. We have too much respect for the character and feelings of the virtuous poor whose misfortunes place them under our care, to subject them to the companionship of the outcasts of society.[20]

Although most patients were not expected to cover the cost of their care, that care was not gratuitous, in either sense of the word: It was neither extravagant nor always free. The historian Charles Rosenberg describes how indigent patients were made to work in exchange for their stays in overcrowded urban hospitals during the nineteenth century, where supplies were inadequate and nurses tore up sheets to use as bandages. Men at Bellevue Hospital were made to row boats on the East River, while pregnant women scrubbed ward floors. In some facilities, patients with venereal diseases who recovered were expected to repay the cost of their care through hospital labor.[21]

By the early decades of the twentieth century, hospitals aimed to entice patients with the means to pay by converting charitable wards into paying wards and private rooms. In addition to private rooms, wealthier patients were offered better food, additional nurses and orderlies, and access to senior physicians.[22] "Voluntary" hospitals, originally built by churches or wealthy local patrons, attempted to attract middle- and upper-class paying patients by highlighting comfortable accommodation alongside access to scientific medical advances. As surgical procedures became more popular, surgical patients of every social class were admitted for their operations.

As hospitals strove to become more hospitable, private physicians with hospital privileges still considered themselves outside the organizational structure, and some fought to ensure they could charge patients separately. One particularly insistent voice in this debate was Gordon Fowler, a surgeon in Brooklyn, New York, who, in 1902, sued eight patients who had not paid separately for his services. While patients and hospital trustees argued physician payments were included in the hospital's charge to patients, Fowler and his attorney prevailed in court. The judge ruled patients could be made to pay separately for services rendered by physicians and surgeons. Due to Fowler's efforts, private-pay patients would have another bill to cover.[23]

Excepting physicians like Fowler, most doctors were reluctant to resort to legal recourse to collect debts. As Baltimore physician Aniel Webster Cathell explained in *The Physician Himself from Graduation to Old Age*, a widely read self-help manual for doctors who lacked "professional tact and business sagacity," first published in 1882, "Medical men who frequently go to law to recover fees generally lose more in the end than they gain; not only because such attempts to recover often prove fruitless, but because they excite prejudice and make influential enemies."[24] Six years later, Cathell's state medical society in Maryland voted down a motion to lobby for the garnishment of wages for medical debt.[25] Both law and custom left medicine forgiving to debtors.

As hospital care became more central to American medicine, the role of charity grew fraught. There were multiple hospital types, with patient populations divided largely along lines of class and worthiness. Private hospital administrators continued to profess a desire to care for the poor, so long as they were without disqualifying vices. They worried aloud about creating a permanent pauper class of unworthy poor who became dependent on charity when they should be working.[26] They left the care of the poor whom they did not wish to admit to public hospitals.

Meanwhile, prominent voices in medicine spoke about free care with deep suspicion. When faced with the custom of charging on a sliding scale, some expressed their frustration with trying to judge patients' financial means, often on the basis of little more than attire and demeanor.[27] Others even expressed disgust the task of caring for the poor. George Shrady, who had served as physician-in-chief of the hospitals of the New York Health Department, wrote in 1897,

It is simply not true that poor people suffer for want of skilled medical attendance. On the contrary, they obtain vastly more than they have a right to expect. . . . Vast sums of money were wasted yearly on worthless and undeserving persons.[28]

Despite this dismissal of the plight of the poor, medical bills did drive patients and their families to despair. One such victim was M. B. Duke, an Atlanta real estate agent and widower with two young children, who in 1912 rented a room in the Hotel Peachtree. There he swallowed enough morphine to end his life. The hotel's owner, a former nurse named Mrs. Monk, heard strange groaning from Duke's room and opened the door. Finding him lethargic and barely breathing, she suspected poisoning. Monk threw a kimono over her nightgown and ran out to buy mustard. When she returned, she shoved it in his mouth, hoping it would induce him to vomit. It did. After purging, Duke eventually roused. He explained he had attempted suicide because he could not hope to repay the medical debts incurred during the treatment of his recently deceased wife.[29]

Plenty of people were denied care at hospitals, as hospital executives maintained it was their right to refuse admission. The historian Beatrix Hoffman recounts a court case that established private hospitals had no duty to provide care. In 1934, the father of 2-year-old Geraldine Crews presented to Baptist Hospital in Birmingham, Alabama. Her throat was coated with a sickly gray film that grew so quickly that she looked like she would soon suffocate. The doctors diagnosed her with diphtheria, a dreaded but treatable bacterial infection. They gave her the antitoxin, but if she was to live she would need other emergent treatments, including supplemental oxygen and endotracheal intubation—that is, a breathing tube to prevent her throat from closing. But due to a hospital policy against admitting patients with potentially contagious diseases, the doctors refused to admit her for this care. Lacking any other options, Geraldine's father carried her out. She died 15 minutes after they returned home. The family sued for wrongful death, but the Alabama state supreme court decided in the hospital's favor. Instead of ruling only on the legality of refusing admission to contagious cases, the justices saw fit to include in their decision a sweeping statement affirming the prerogatives of private hospitals: "Private hospitals owed [the] public no duty to accept any patient not desired by [the] hospital, and were not required to assign reason for refusal to accept."[30] For decades thereafter, hospitals and courts would cite this decision in justifying all manner of refusals to deliver care.

Even as state and local grants to private hospitals overtook charitable donations as the largest source of funding in the 1930s, this aid came with no obligation to provide care to the indigent.[31] Late in life, former President Harry Truman remembered that as a county court judge in Missouri during the 1920s and 1930s he "saw people turned away from hospitals to die because they had no money for treatment."[32] Black Americans had even fewer options for medical treatment. Until the mid-1960s, hospitals across much of the country were segregated by race, so Black patients had to seek care at the relatively few Black hospitals or in segregated wards. Black activists and even mainstream publications documented frequent instances of hospitals refusing care to critically ill patients on account of race.[33]

To ensure payment from patients who were allowed through the door, hospitals increased their collection efforts. During the 1930s, patients were, upon discharge, escorted to the cashier's desk to pay for their stays. Some hospitals joined together to form collection agencies to seek payments from those who did not pay at discharge.[34] Patients in arrears could expect to receive dunning letters, which were ever-more-threatening notices demanding past-due payment.[35]

Charity-care remained a part of the hospital's stated mission, but in contrast to their nineteenth-century predecessors, hospitals and private physicians relied increasingly on third-party payers. By the mid-twentieth century, private health insurance was the major source of hospital revenues. Insurance benefits accounted for 64 percent of all nongovernmental payments for hospital care in 1960.[36] By 1964, 47 million Americans held major medical coverage insurance policies.[37] And, beginning in 1950, the federal government began to provide grants to states to pay for some of the care given to people receiving public assistance. Whereas charity cases accounted for the majority of hospitalizations until the early twentieth century, by 1953, voluntary hospitals claimed that only 3.5 percent of their total patient charges were uncollectible, while private for-profit hospitals claimed a figure of 5.9 percent and government hospitals 6.2 percent. Hospitals did not report how many patients were offered charity-care, and which were sent to collections.[38] With the growth of private insurance, both physicians and patients became less involved in the process of billing and collections.

The federal role in paying for the care of the indigent increased again with the passage of Medicaid and Medicare in 1965, which covered some of America's poor and a large portion of the medical expenses for Americans older than age 65 years, respectively. During the ceremony when he signed these programs into law, President Lyndon Johnson proclaimed an end to the era of unbearable medical bills for America's seniors:

> No longer will older Americans be denied the healing miracle of modern medicine. No longer will illness crush and destroy the savings that they have so carefully put away over a lifetime so that they might enjoy dignity in their later years.[39]

The enactment of Medicare and Medicaid did mark a major shift in American health policy and rapidly afforded a measure of financial protection to a large portion of America's most vulnerable patients. As seniors were rapidly enrolled in Medicare, the percentage of uninsured declined at a rate that would not be matched until the period immediately following the expansion of Medicaid eligibility under the terms of the Affordable Care Act in 2014 (Figure 1.1). Later analyses would find that Americans are much less likely to accrue new medical debt after turning 65 years old, when they become eligible for Medicare; this effect is even larger if they are uninsured prior to Medicare eligibility.[40]

The enactment of these laws did not, however, stop a broader shift away from the model of hospitals as almshouses. The shift to third-party financing by public and private insurers decreased the importance of

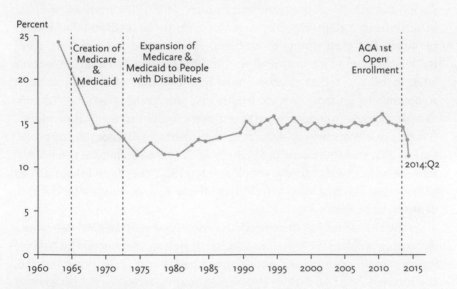

Figure 1.1: Uninsured rate in the United States, 1964–2014.
Source: Jason Furman and Matt Fielder, "2014 Has Seen Largest Coverage Gains in Four Decades, Putting the Uninsured Rate at or Near Historic Lows," Obama White House Blog, December 18, 2014.

charitable donations in hospital budgets and led to a more wholesale acceptance in the public mind of the hospital as an enterprise in search of patients whose care would be paid for. In a 1978 federal court decision, a judge in Michigan gave voice to this sentiment: "The modern hospital, whether operated by a city, a church, or a group of private investors, is essentially a business."[41]

The passage of Medicare and Medicaid did not eliminate the problem of medical debt, particularly for those who did not reside on "islands of social citizenship," as Gabriel Winant termed the private and public insurance protections afforded to some, though never all, Americans starting in the mid-twentieth century.[42] Before the rise of private health insurance and easy access to consumer credit, people in debt to their doctor might turn to better-off friends, family, or mutual aid societies to help repay. If they did not have any of these resources, working-class patients sometimes turned to loan sharks who charged interest as high as 20 percent for funds to repay their debts.[43] During the Great Depression, American businesses avoided borrowing, so commercial banks sought out new opportunities for profitable lending. When they began to offer relatively low-interest personal loans to middle-class customers, as the Manufacturers Trust Company and National City Bank did during the mid-1930s, they discovered that medical and dental bills accounted for between 20 and 30 percent of the costs their borrowers planned to cover.[44]

Medical care was the source of a significant and growing financial burden during the middle of the twentieth century. In a 1930 study of personal bankruptcies in Kentucky, 31 percent of filers listed medical bills on their petitions. But even among those filers who included medical debt, medical bills accounted for only 19.4 percent of total debt.[45] A quarter-century later, in 1954, a report commissioned by a coalition of health insurance companies to promote private health insurance estimated that 7.5 million households (roughly one in seven) were in debt to medical providers. A family in arrears held an average medical debt of $121; accounting for inflation, this was equivalent to $1,310 in 2022.[46] Researchers at the Federal Reserve had arrived at similar conclusions in 1952; they found that families with young children were particularly likely to owe money to doctors, dentists, or hospitals.[47]

In the second half of the twentieth century, even as medical debt was a worsening problem for American families, hospitals successfully lobbied for less demanding regulations around their charity-care obligations. In 1956, the Internal Revenue Service (IRS) ruled that in exchange for tax exemption, a nonprofit hospital had to provide charity-care "to the extent of its financial ability for those not able to pay for service rendered."[48] Although the IRS did not specify how much was sufficient, its rule was more than a paper tiger. When a charity-care program accounted for less than 5 percent of a hospital's gross revenues, auditing agents usually recommended denial or revocation of its tax-exempt status.[49] But after the passage of Medicare and Medicaid in 1965, hospitals pushed for a new standard of tax exemption. One of their main contentions ("almost hilarious, in retrospect, for its inaccuracy," according to legal historian John Colombo[50]) was that with the rise of private insurance and the enactment of government insurance for the poor and the elderly, there was much not need for hospital-funded charity-care. Hospital administrators also questioned exactly how much charity-care they were expected to provide. What, precisely, did it mean for a hospital to provide charity-care "to the extent of its financial ability"?[51]

In response, Robert Bromberg, a Brooklyn-born, Columbia-educated, 34-year-old staff attorney at the IRS, worked to develop a new standard for tax exemption—one that moved hospitals far from the almshouse tradition. Released in 1969 without public comment, this new rule replaced the 1956 "charity care standard" with what became known as a "community benefit standard." This rule asserted that even if the indigent were excluded from care, hospitals could justify their charitable purpose through work toward the "promotion of health" for the general benefit of the community. Bromberg echoed hospital executives' claims when he argued that the enactment of Medicare and Medicaid and the spread of private health insurance "diminished the amount of free care needed." He dismissed the old expectation "that the charitable hospital primarily concern itself with the poor," because "the hospital as an almshouse disappeared over a century ago."[52] In place of this "anachronism," he set forth a new, more minimal definition of a charitable hospital eligible for tax exemption: "The open emergency room and the willingness to take all paying patients . . . are the existential requirements imposed to insure that the charitable hospital is responsive to the community's needs."[53]

Bromberg's rule allowed hospitals to demonstrate fitness for tax exemption by having a community board and by treating Medicare and Medicaid patients. A subsequent ruling did require tax-exempt hospitals to do more than treat paying patients, but charity-care was not the only activity that could satisfy the IRS. Spending surplus funds on medical research, teaching, and new patient care facilities could also demonstrate community benefit.[54] Thus, following the 1969 ruling, care of the poor was no longer the main criterion by which tax exemption would be determined. The leadership of the American Hospital Association so appreciated Bromberg's reasoning that upon his departure from the IRS for a more lucrative career in corporate law, they hired him as their Special Tax Counsel.[55]

Even as the IRS was paying less attention to poor patients, some politicians took up the issue of medical debt. In 1971, Senator Edward Kennedy of Massachusetts held a series of public hearings of the Senate Health Subcommittee. Kennedy subsequently wrote *In Critical Condition*, a book based on the hearings. In a chapter provocatively titled "Businessmen or Healers?" he recounted the outrages related in testimonies from everyday Americans:

> We've heard stories of people who are turned away by hospitals unless they can make deposits or can show evidence of insurance; people ejected from . . . their hospital rooms because their insurance was inadequate or had run out . . . people who are hounded by collection agencies that buy the hospitals' and doctors' "bad debts" or get a percentage of what they collect; people who are forced into bankruptcy by their medical bills and forced afterwards to pay before they are treated.[56]

Around this time, journalists also took note of the rising tide of medical debt. The lack of access to care that stemmed from both stringent criteria for Medicaid coverage and the paucity of charity-care was evident to the journalist Daniel Schorr when he conducted interviews for his 1970 book and television special, both titled *Don't Get Sick in America*. In Chicago, a doctor reported that whenever he tried to admit one of his indigent patients to any hospital other than government-run Cook County, administrators would complain bitterly that he was sending them "another welfare patient."[57]

In Lee County, Arkansas, where Black residents were losing their meager livings as tenant farmers to mechanized cotton cultivation, Schorr learned how readily doctors refused care to people without cash on hand. One resident recounted taking a friend to the doctor:

> Before she put a hand on her, she said, "Do you have any money, honey?" And the lady told her she had some. The doctor said she wanted to know where she was goin' to get the money from. If you ain't got no money, you don't see no doctor. You just have to suffer it out.[58]

The doctor disputed the story, telling Schorr she had never turned anyone away for want of money. She did argue that "the exchange of money is necessary to establish the proper relationship between doctor and patient."[59] What is notable about this story, though, is that it was still normal for conversations over payment to be had directly between doctor and patient.

As Chapter 2 shows, this social relation would not be maintained for long, as debts came to be transacted more impersonally.

In 1972, an act of desperation spurred in part by medical debt produced splashy headlines. Heinrick von George was an unemployed insurance salesman living in the Boston suburb of Brockton who was deep in debt after his 8-year-old son Early had to undergo surgery at Massachusetts General Hospital to repair a congenital heart defect. Von George had a desperate plan to find the money. He left his home, telling his wife he was going to look for a job. He drove to Albany, New York, where he boarded a plane bound for New York City. Thirty minutes after takeoff, he pulled out a gun and announced he was hijacking the plane. He showed containers wrapped around his chest and claimed it was a bomb. He demanded the plane land at Westchester County Airport, where he allowed the 42 passengers to disembark but kept one of the flight attendants as a hostage. There he collected $200,000 ransom before demanding to be flown to Poughkeepsie.[60]

Von George's plan was eerily similar to a ploy executed successfully the previous year by D. B. Cooper, who had hijacked a plane in Portland, Oregon, and secured a $200,000 ransom during a stop in Seattle. After the plane took off again, Cooper donned a parachute and jumped out of the plane, never to be heard from again. Von George was not so successful. After his plane landed in Poughkeepsie, he pushed the flight attendant into a waiting car and tried to drive away. An agent from the Federal Bureau of Investigation walked up to the vehicle and shot and killed von George. His bomb turned out to be two canteens filled with water, and the gun was a blank starter pistol.[61]

Anecdotes, sometimes sensational ones, remained the mainstay of reporting about medical debt for most of the twentieth century. Meanwhile, legal and public health journals published precious little on the problem. Those few articles that did venture into the subject found medical bills to be, at most, one kind of debt among many that consumers struggled to repay. Legal scholars Teresa Sullivan, Elizabeth Warren, and Jay Lawrence Westbrook published a study of bankruptcy filers from 10 federal court districts in 1981 across three states: Illinois, Pennsylvania, and Texas. They found that although more than half of the debtors listed medical debt in their files, such debts were not a primary driver of bankruptcy. Most of these filers had "more modest medical debts," while "at most only 1% to 2% of the debtors in bankruptcy are demonstrably there because of catastrophic medical losses."[62] Although they suspected that reliance on court records might result in an underestimation of the role of medical debt, the results did suggest that mid-century social protections, including

Medicare, Medicaid, and private insurance, had provided a bulwark against the worst effects of medical debt.

That did not last for long. Twenty years later, Elizabeth Warren and Amelia Warren Tyagi found that the number of families declaring bankruptcy who had experienced health-related financial stress had increased more than 2,000 percent.[63] Medical debts, and the intensity of efforts to collect them, were about to explode.

CHAPTER 2

No Mercy

Debt in the Late Twentieth Century

Pay it I will to the end—
Until the grave, my friend,
Gives me a true release—
Gives me the clasp of peace.

—Paul Laurence Dunbar, "The Debt"

Medical debts have long spurred people to desperate acts: theft, suicide, plane hijacking. But the modern era of pay-up-or-else health financing and aggressive debt collection began in earnest during the last two decades of the twentieth century, as threats to their own survival made hospitals less financially forgiving toward their patients. During this era, the growth in both federal and state government spending on Medicare and Medicaid slowed dramatically, and the effects were compounded by rising health care costs and reined-in reimbursements by private insurance, all of which led hospitals to adopt aggressive collection tactics to get patients to pay their bills.

During the late twentieth century, America's nascent and incomplete welfare state was on the ropes. Recession and the apparent failure of Keynesian economics during the 1970s played a role in this turning of the tide. Policymakers were also inspired by the market fundamentalism of economists Milton Friedman and Friedrich Hayek. Some showed a zeal to demonize the poor, as when in 1976 then-presidential candidate Ronald Reagan decried welfare recipients living large off the public dole. Mayors, governors, members of Congress, and presidents advocated for a series of cost-cutting measures including new restrictions on cash welfare benefits as well as decreased funding for affordable housing and relief for the homeless. In cities and states throughout the country, these measures were part of a new orthodoxy.[1] Some liberal politicians foresaw this ideological shift and even warned of the impact on medical debts. In his acceptance speech for the vice-presidential nomination at the Democratic National Convention in 1980, incumbent Vice President Walter Mondale warned of a coming transformation, which he saw as anathema to American values: "Most Americans believe that no family should be impoverished by medical debts when tragic illness strikes—but not Ronald Reagan."[2]

Reagan won that election in a landslide, a victory that ushered in a wave of welfare-state retrenchment.[3] Two elements of his administration's cost-cutting proved particularly painful for health care institutions. The first involved a change in provider payments for Medicare, the government program for the elderly. In 1983, Medicare moved from retrospectively reimbursing all "reasonable costs" (a definition left largely up to hospitals) to prospective payments set by the federal government based on predetermined rates for "diagnosis related groups."[4] The Reagan administration and prominent Democrats in Congress aimed to use this measure to control rapidly rising Medicare spending. The hospital lobby, although not pleased with this solution, found it preferable to a cost-cutting measure passed by Congress the previous year that threatened to institute even stricter limits on reimbursement.[5]

The second change was a sharp deceleration in spending growth on Medicaid, the government program for the poor. Medicaid had, like Medicare, been required by law to meet hospitals' "reasonable costs" since the program's enactment in 1965. But in 1981, new federal regulations freed Medicaid from this requirement. States quickly took the opportunity to put the brakes on Medicaid spending. By 1987, in an attempt to limit costs, 34 states had instituted prospective payment in their Medicaid programs. In addition, new restrictions in Medicaid eligibility led to a decrease in the number of people in the program, from 22 million in 1974 to 21 million in 1984, even as the number of people living below the federal poverty level increased from 23 million to 34 million during that time.[6] The share of poor and near-poor covered by Medicaid decreased from 63 percent in 1975 to 46 percent in 1985.[7]

While state and federal Medicaid funding had grown on an inflation-adjusted basis of 6 percent per year during the 1970s, in the first half of the 1980s this rate fell by almost half, to 3.4 percent.[8] Congress did direct states to give additional funds to hospitals that served a disproportionate share of low-income patients, and provided federal allotments for the same purpose, but these payments were, in most states, both insufficient to meet the scale of the need and inequitably distributed among hospitals.[9]

This spending slowdown occurred while medical technology continued to become more intensive and more expensive. As a result, the care of patients covered by Medicaid and Medicare became a source of net losses for hospitals. Between 1980 and 1990, Medicare payment-to-cost ratios fell from 0.96 to 0.89, and Medicaid payment-to-cost ratios fell from 0.91 to 0.80.[10] In addition, due to the severe restrictions on Medicaid eligibility in many states, there was a significant population of uninsured patients who continued to account for the majority of hospitals' uncompensated care costs.[11]

During the 1980s, hospitals were able to make up for the slowdown in government payments by increasing private insurance reimbursements. But by the early 1990s, private insurers were no longer willing to make up the shortfall; they refused to reimburse significantly in excess of charges for their own patients.[12] This was due, in large part, to the rise of managed care. Prior to the 1980s, the majority of American workers were enrolled in indemnity ("fee-for-service") plans, with relatively generous reimbursements given to any provider the patient chose to see. However, as insurance premiums rose, employers seeking to control their costs turned to managed care plans such as health maintenance organizations. These insurance plans reimbursed only those providers who agreed to the prices they offered, which were up to 30 percent lower than the older indemnity plans for high-tech services.[13] Patients faced huge out-of-pocket payments if they sought care outside these networks, while hospitals and physicians received less for care they provided to managed care patients. The plans were unpopular with patients and health care providers, in part because they required the insurance company's permission for specialist referrals, imaging, hospitalizations, and other decisions traditionally made by physicians. Crucially, because they charged lower premiums than traditional insurance, they did allow employers to rein in spending on employee health insurance benefits. This fact drove a massive shift: Whereas in 1980 more than 90 percent of privately insured individuals were enrolled in unmanaged indemnity insurance, by 2000 more than 90 percent were in managed care.[14]

For President Reagan and other opponents of the welfare state, discomforting many low-income Americans was the point. There were, they argued, unworthy poor who needed to learn to provide for themselves. As President Reagan put it when he was asked to explain his antipathy to Medicare and Medicaid spending at a 1981 press conference, "The main goal of any of these reductions is still aimed at correcting those abuses that . . . allow people who do not have a real need that justifies their imposing on their fellow citizens for sustenance."[15]

Both patients and hospitals suffered under this new regime. According to the American Hospital Association, the costs of uncompensated care more than doubled between 1980 and 1984.[16] (Uncompensated care was a figure that, at the time, combined charity-care offered by the hospital and bad debt—charges that hospitals attempted to collect but could not.) This burden was not shared equally by all hospitals. In 1983, public hospitals' uncompensated care as a share of revenues was more than twice as high as that of private nonprofit hospitals and more than three times higher than that of investor-owned hospitals.[17]

Many public and private nonprofit facilities did not survive. What happened to hospitals in the 1980s very nearly met the literal definition of decimation, as 9.7 percent closed for good.[18] Other struggling hospitals were bought out by investor-owned, for-profit hospital chains. In 1986, the Hospital Corporation of America, an investor-owned hospital chain based in Tennessee, already owned more than 30 hospitals previously owned by county governments.[19] By the mid-1980s, nearly half of hospitals in Florida, Texas, Nevada, and New Mexico were for-profit institutions.[20]

In this environment, both private nonprofit and for-profit hospitals began to view charity-care more as an unaffordable luxury than as a pursuit central to their missions. In 1987, Congressman Ralph Regula, a Republican from Ohio, described the trend with the language of a diplomat: "Limited by finite payments, providers have been driven into a de facto system of allocating services based to some extent on criteria other than patient need."[21] The reality was more cruel. Private hospitals took to "dumping" patients, demanding up-front payment for care and then sending patients who failed the "wallet biopsy" to the few remaining and overburdened public facilities. The *Chicago Tribune* reported that immediately after Medicaid cuts in Illinois in the summer of 1981, these euphemistically named "economic transfers" to Cook County Hospital, a public facility, more than tripled. Some private hospitals provided no treatment to these patients before sending them away: Trauma victims were transferred while bleeding to death, and pregnant women were put in ambulances as they were about to deliver.[22]

This practice was galling to doctors and advocates for the poor. In 1984, David Himmelstein, a medical resident at Highland Hospital in Oakland, California, saw that many patients were being transferred to his hospital for unclear reasons. After carefully examining medical charts, he and his colleagues found that 97 percent of patients who were transferred from a private hospital to a public hospital in Oakland were either uninsured or publicly insured. Only one out of the 103 transfers had been justified on medical grounds, whereas 11 were explicitly transferred for inability to pay.[23]

Following this study, Eugene Barnes, a 32-year-old Black man, died after being stabbed by an assailant and then being refused treatment at a hospital in Oakland. Representative Pete Stark, a Democrat representing the Oakland area, responded to these revelations by writing the Emergency Medical Treatment and Active Labor Act (EMTALA). This law, passed as an amendment to a budget bill in 1986, required hospitals that accept Medicare funds to provide a medical screening exam as well as treatment to stabilize any emergent medical condition for patients who presented to their emergency departments.[24]

Although EMTALA aimed to ensure a modicum of care in emergencies, hospitals complained that this new mandate came without funding to help them implement it. EMTALA became a byword for the threadbare right to medical care in the United States, but it provided no protection against financial ruin for either hospitals or patients. Hospitals adopted explicit limits on the charity-care they would provide, no matter how many needy patients presented to their emergency departments. In 1990, at Raritan Bay Medical Center in New Jersey, patients were made to jump through hoop after hoop to qualify for charity-care. The application patients had to submit included earnings receipts, tax returns, bank statements, and utility bills, and a family of four would qualify for a discount only if they earned less than $24,000 per year—less than twice the federal poverty level.[25] At other hospitals, registrars were told to demand that non-emergency patients provide deposits, in the form of cash or credit card, prior to admission.[26]

Still, hospital executives bemoaned a "tide of bad debt," including both unpaid deductibles and co-payments as well as bills owed by the uninsured. Such debts increased from 3.7 percent of gross hospital revenues in the first quarter of 1988 to 4.3 percent in the first quarter of 1991.[27] By 2001, a review of bankruptcy cases in Indiana found that 35 percent of filers said they owed at least $1,000 to medical providers, with some owing six-figure sums.[28] Hospitals had taken out debts of their own, spurred by the low interest rates of the 1990s and the promise of high returns in the stock market.[29] But when patients' unpaid debts became theirs, hospitals faced risks to their own credit ratings and feared triggering bond covenants with creditors.

In response, some hospitals found new ways to pass along the financial burden to patients. Whereas patients had traditionally been allowed to work out payment plans over years, or pay a steep discount, now they were given less lenience. In Poughkeepsie, New York, in 1991, Vassar Brothers

Hospital ended its installment program for low-income patients and instead compelled patients with planned hospital stays to apply for commercial loans from Barclays Bank to ensure up-front payment.[30] Other hospitals issued their own private-label, high-interest credit cards that could be used to purchase services only with them, or they had patients take out consumer lines of credit with a preferred bank.[31]

Even as financial assistance waned and tactics to ensure payment grew more harsh, uninsured patients were charged more for hospital care than anyone else. Through at least the 1960s, hospitals based their "chargemaster," or list prices, on costs plus a markup of approximately 10 percent. But beginning in the 1980s, hospitals tried to make up for constrained revenues and prospective payments from Medicare and Medicaid by increasing list prices to shift more costs to private insurers. In response, managed care companies and other private insurers used their market power to negotiate discounts with hospitals. Seeking to strengthen their position in these negotiations, hospitals increased their list prices still further.[32]

This contest between hospitals and insurance companies actually affected the uninsured the most because they were the ones who were actually made to pay these list prices. As hospital financing expert Gerard Anderson has argued, "The only people paying full charges are those with limited or no bargaining power."[33] By 2004, uninsured patients were charged 2.5 times more for hospital care than those with private insurance and 3 times more than those with Medicare.[34]

In another ironic turn, by increasing the prices they charged the uninsured, hospitals could make it seem like they were being more charitable—because they used their list prices to calculate the amount of charity-care they provided, resulting in a vast overestimation of this community benefit in reports submitted to the Internal Revenue Service to justify their tax-exempt status.[35] While hospitals used high charges to inflate the public's opinion of their charitable works, those actually in need of charity bore the brunt of inflated costs.

Hospital spokespeople repeatedly insisted that no one actually paid these charges and that low-income patients could apply for charity-care. But, as discussed later, hospitals were often less than eager to publicize charity-care policies to patients, and applying was not easy. Even when applications were completed, many were denied. Even if a patient was granted a discount, it was based on the inflated charges, so they could easily end up paying more than government or private insurers. And when patients' debts were handed over to collectors, the charges they would be hounded to pay were not based on the actual cost the hospital paid to provide that care but, rather, on these high list prices.

This was an era of much brainstorming about creative and coercive ways to wrangle payments from vulnerable patients. For non-emergent care, hospitals and physicians' offices routinely required up-front payments for elective procedures, encouraged uninsured patients to seek care elsewhere, or refused to see patients with unpaid bills.[36] Despite the dictates of EMTALA, hospital administrators still sought ways to wring more money out of patients presenting to the emergency room.[37]

Although some patients could be induced to pay up-front, hospitals relied, most of all, on debt collection. Health care institutions had run in-house collection departments since the 1930s, but these departments tended to work slowly, leaving bad debts on their books for years, even decades. Executives in billing departments once believed their role was to ensure that the patient–physician relationship was not embittered by their practices. "It's certainly not our intent to leave a bad taste in their mouths," explained Bill Fisher, assistant administrator for finance at Holy Family in Spokane, Washington, in 1992.[38] But this was no longer the main concern for hospital finance executives in the new era, when hospitals worked to settle debts more quickly, and the aims of billing departments changed. At the Halifax Hospital Medical Center in Daytona, Florida, staff received bonuses when collections surpassed targets.[39]

Private insurers had their own interests in seeing hospitals beef up collection efforts. As Donald Cohodes, executive director of policy for the Blue Cross and Blue Shield Association, wrote in 1986,

> Hospitals that fail to vigorously pursue their bad debt population are contributors to the problem. After all, the real effect of debt forgiveness by hospitals is to decrease incentives to purchase health insurance. Why buy health insurance if it is not necessary to pay for it?[40]

Seeking to ensure that patients were made to pay for their care, Cohodes advised hospitals to push more patients to use credit cards to settle debts.

The biggest shift came when health care institutions decided they would no longer handle debt collection on their own. By the 1980s and 1990s, when patients did not pay their bills, hospitals and physicians' offices were more willing to hand the collection process over to more rough-and-tumble third-party collection agencies.[41] As the ranks of the underinsured and the uninsured continued to grow, hospitals sought out firms that could ensure prompt repayment. By 1993, the American Collectors Association (later, ACA International) claimed that hospitals were the source of more business than any other industry.[42] Yet even as providers turned more bills over to collection agencies, they expressed some trepidation. Fisher, the executive at Holy Family in Spokane, said collection agencies were a "necessary evil" and added, ruefully, "They're not exactly a public relations arm. You want to get one that doesn't hurt you."[43]

A typical pattern emerged in private practices and hospitals. Between 2 and 6 months after patients failed to pay, the practice would assign the debt to a collection agency on a contingency basis. These agencies specialized in contacting patients in ways designed to make them pay as expeditiously as possible. The first, and oldest, method was through dunning letters, which chastised the borrower with increasingly aggressive language. If those did not work, the agency escalated to phone calls and even home visits. For small bills, if the agency did not want to spend money on phone calls, they sometimes reported the debt to credit bureaus without contacting the debtor. This step, known as "parking," was intended to prompt the debtor call the collector directly—after they tried to apply for a loan, a job, or a new apartment and received word that their credit was not as good as they thought or when they happened to look at their credit report or FICO score.[44] If the agency was able to collect a debt, it would keep as much as 40 percent of the money collected and send the rest back to the hospital. Debts that remained unpaid after an agreed period, often a year, would revert back to the hospital.[45]

Patients and legal advocates complained that hospitals did not adequately screen patients to ensure poor patients were not sent to collections. As one Nebraska woman who faced thousands of dollars in bills after an admission for a bleeding stomach ulcer explained, "The hospital always says, 'Well, if you're indigent or whatever, they'll help you.' But they never do."[46] In 1999, a survey of low-income adults in Pittsburgh, Pennsylvania, found that 44 percent of respondents had outstanding medical debt, and 31 percent had been referred to collections in the past year; people were more likely to have been referred if they were Black, were uninsured, had an income less than $750 per month, or had no usual source of medical care.[47] A national survey 2 years later found that among the uninsured, who were overwhelmingly low-income, 36 percent had been contacted by a collection agency for unpaid medical bills in the past year.[48]

Not everyone viewed this situation as a cause for concern. Debt collection was big business, and it was getting bigger. In 2004, three-fourths of the member agencies of ACA International collected health care debt.[49] In 2006, the research firm Kaulkin Ginsberg estimated that America's 6,000 hospitals generated $129 billion in bad debt every year, of which $42.6 billion was assigned to debt collection agencies or sold to debt buyers.[50]

Whereas hospitals were relatively eager to assign their debts to third-party collectors, they were, for a time, more reluctant to sell them outright.

Hospital executives and physicians had long feared that giving up control of their accounts by selling debts would bring negative publicity. "'Hospital auctions bad debt to collection agencies' doesn't read well in the press," explained Dan Rode, director of policy and government relations at the Healthcare Financial Management Association, in 1993.[51] For decades, as other forms of consumer debt were securitized and sold on financial markets, medical debt was handled differently. Even when it was assigned to debt collectors, hospitals still held ultimate ownership over the debt, and therefore over the tactics employed to collect it. There was still some financial link, however slight, between the doctors and nurses caring for the patient and the patient faced with the bill.

But by the 1990s, some hospitals had grown tired enough of trying to collect their own debts that they sold them outright. In 1992, Principal Residential Advisor (PRA), a Florida-based subsidiary of the insurance and investment management company Principal Financial Group, started offering hospitals the opportunity to auction their bad debt to its list of 1,800 collection agencies. Instead of assigning debts on a contingency basis, these auctions promised hospitals guaranteed payments from debt collectors, which would in turn try to collect as much as possible from patients. Because collection agencies were taking on all the risk of debt collection, they were only willing to pay a small portion of the face value of the bad debts owed to hospitals. In its first sale, PRA sold $1.1 million in debt owed to Ed Fraser Memorial Hospital, a public hospital just south of the Florida–Georgia state line, for $52,000, or 4.7 cents on the dollar, to United Asset Recovery, a collection agency in Ohio. The hospital made only $39,000 because it had to pay PRA's 25 percent fee for brokering the transaction.[52] Still, Dennis Markso, Fraser's chief financial officer (CFO), claimed the sale was necessary. Given the facility's recent budget deficits, selling debt was "just one of the things we're doing to try to turn this hospital around."[53]

PRA's move was noteworthy not only because it helped forge a new market for distressed hospital receivables but also because it marked the tentative start of a new, more aggressive chapter in the history of medical debt collection. Yet most hospital executives were still wary about selling debt. The debt-buying industry did not have a sparkling reputation, for good reason. A few months after PRA brokered the debt sale between the Florida hospital and the Ohio agency, a different debt collector was in the news. The Securities and Exchange Commission charged Stephen Hoffenberg—the brash, well-connected owner of the New York-based Towers Financial Corporation—with running a Ponzi scheme. Hoffenberg had sold bonds to credulous investors, promising high rates of return. He then claimed that he could deliver huge profits by successfully collecting on consumer debts, including hospitals' bad debts, for which he had paid mere cents on the dollar. In its financial statements, the company lied about its recovery rates, thereby inflating the value of its assets.[54] Criminal charges followed, and Hoffenberg claimed that the fraud was the work of his young business partner, Jeffrey Epstein. Epstein was never charged for this crime, while Hoffenberg was found guilty and sentenced to 20 years in prison.[55]

Over time, the tide of executive opinion moved in favor of increasing revenues, regardless of the consequences. Hospital executives were awash in a rising sentiment that medical care was a commodity, to be bought and sold like any other. As the physician and social theorist Richard Gunderman observed in a 1998 essay,

> Ours is an era in which the jargon of the business schools plays a growing role in the discourse of medicine. Health care is increasingly regarded as a business, the physician as a businessman, and the coin of commerce serves increasingly as the common currency of medical discourse. Patients have become "health care consumers," "clients," or even "customers."[56]

Debt buyers were beneficiaries of this shift. Still, they sought to allay hospital executives' concerns over reputational risks by associating themselves with respectable figures. The advisory board of Senex Services Corporation, a debt collection firm founded in 1998 and based in Indianapolis, Indiana, included former Vice President Dan Quayle.[57]

During the late 1990s and early 2000s, small sales did occur, while debt buyers eagerly anticipated a gold rush. In this era of financial innovation, they touted medical debt as a profitable new instrument. "It's the place to be," promised Patrick Bracken, marketing director of Performance Financial Corporation, in 2000, noting that at his firm recovery rates for medical debts exceeded those for credit card debt and other forms of consumer debt.[58] Senex trumpeted an agreement it had signed with the University HealthSystem Consortium in 2004 to be the preferred buyer of debt from 91 academic medical centers.[59] But the rush had not yet begun. In 2004, while total medical debt in the United States was estimated at $120 billion, only $1 billion in health care debt sales had been publicly disclosed.[60]

Two years later, the moment had arrived. Tenet Healthcare, one of the largest for-profit hospital chains in the country, sold $1.2 billion in debt for $16 million.[61] The bonanza was not limited to investor-owned hospitals. When a large public hospital put its bad debt up for sale, a reporter asked why it was not assigning the debt to collection agencies to retain more control over the tactics employed. The CFO was defiant: "We're done with that.

From now on, we're going to sell the paper at 180 days. We're not going to wait around for our money."[62]

Hospital executives were eager to offload debt even though they would have to sell it for pennies on the dollar. After all, internal hospital collection departments tended to collect only 6 to 9 cents on the dollar from uninsured patients. In 2006, a Texas nonprofit hospital sold 1,656 accounts and a face value of $157,000 to debt buyer Medicorp for $14,000. In other words, Medicorp paid 8.9 cents on the dollar.[63] Rates for out-of-pocket payments from insured patients could be much higher, as much as 50 cents on the dollar.[64] Accounts that been already been "worked" by a collection agency might sell for a quarter-penny on the dollar. Other older accounts might sell for more, particularly if they had not been delinquent for long or if the hospital allowed the debt buyer to take patients to court.[65]

Early buyers of medical debt faced nagging questions about political and legal risks. Would new laws limit their ability to collect? By the early 2000s, politicians such as Minnesota Attorney General Mike Hatch, a Democrat with his sights on the governor's office, and Representative James Greenwood, a Republican from Pennsylvania, were garnering headlines by holding press conferences and hearings to expose aggressive hospital collection tactics and proposing additional regulations. As later chapters will show, labor unions and other activists were also agitating for an end to these debt collection tactics.

Even with these concerns, corporations saw promise in the growing market for medical debt. Large publicly traded companies, including Portfolio Recovery Associates and Acceptance Capital Corporation, announced new units devoted to buying medical receivables.[66] Cargill, a Minnesota-based agricultural company and the largest private company in the United States, was best known in financial markets for grain dealing.[67] But between 2002 and 2007, it purchased more than $7 billion in health care receivables.[68]

Encore Capital Group, a publicly traded company that was fast becoming one of the largest buyers and collectors of consumer debt in the United States, started its medical debt-buying business in 2005, when it spent $4.27 million to buy debt with a face value of $274 million. The company partnered with the Receivables Management Bureau, a collection agency specializing in medical debt. Brandon Black, Encore's president, called medical debt buying "a huge opportunity for us."[69] To finance its mission to "build the leading company in the distressed consumer space," Encore turned to big banks and claimed to have secured $200 million in capital, including $35 million from J. P. Morgan, $30 million from Bank of America, $30 million from the Bank of Scotland, and $15 million from Citibank.[70]

There was no single platform that hosted most exchanges of medical debt or consumer debt generally. CFOs sold debt through personal contacts with debt collection professionals—connections forged through conferences, networking events, or cold calls. But the early 1990s brought some order to the process of buying and selling this "paper," as it was called in the industry. This order came as a by-product of another scandal, the Savings and Loan crisis that had been triggered by deregulation and fraud and had resulted in a bailout. This left the US Treasury holding more than $500 billion in consumer debt. This massive supply of debt spurred a more systematic way of pricing bad debts, which allowed buyers, large and small, to enter a market once widely viewed as too uncertain for serious investors.[71]

Some large-scale buyers had huge in-house collection departments; others outsourced collection on a contingency basis to other agencies. But many collection agencies were short-lived, tiny, fly-by-night operations, with low-paid employees working on quotas.[72] Of the estimated 6,500 companies that bought debt outright, rather than operating solely on contingency, 95 percent had less than $8 million in revenue in 2005.[73] These smaller agencies could prove desperately aggressive in their tactics because failure to collect could lead to their own bankruptcies.[74]

The structure of the industry was a breeding ground for abuse. Collectors used a variety of tactics to cajole patients to pay up. Although the Fair Debt Collection Practices Act of 1978 prohibited third-party agencies from certain abusive activities, such as late-night phone calls, abusive language, or telling other individuals about the debt, blatant violations of these rules were incredibly common. The Federal Trade Commission fielded reports from Americans of obscene language, racial and ethnic slurs, or harassing phone calls at work. Collectors could be creative in exploiting debtors' vulnerabilities. There was the immigrant who was threatened with deportation, the elderly man who was urged to sell his glass eye, and the down-on-his-luck debtor who was told he was worth more dead than alive.[75] Richard Bell, one veteran debt collector, said that in his office, reducing the debtor on the other end of the telephone line to tears was "a badge of honor." During such calls, the agent put the caller on speakerphone so that everyone could hear the sobs.[76]

The aim of these tactics was to secure prompt payment. But collectors knew that debtors rarely had spare money lying around to pay their bills. To draw blood from a stone, the debtor often had to be compelled to submit to an even more precarious financial position. They were encouraged to trade one kind of debt for another, by using high-interest credit cards or payday loans, if only to stay the tirade.[77] For the debtor, this desperate move offered little respite: Credit card companies reported delinquent debt to credit bureaus even more regularly than did medical debt collectors, and credit card debt was more disreputable to future lenders. Thus, as a result of putting a medical bill on a credit card, debtors might be relegated to a future of credit that included only subprime and predatory loans. Their medical woes had metastasized to every other facet of their financial lives.[78] As Melissa Jacoby, professor of law at the University of North Carolina and an expert on medical bankruptcies, explained, "One expensive trip to a hospital, followed by zealous collection and reporting, can bring about a host of unexpected negative effects."[79]

There is, in most Americans' minds, a safety net of charity-care designed to spare the most vulnerable patients from the clutches of such financial predation. Yet even when patients were eligible for charity-care by hospitals' stringent rules, the onus remained on them to apply for it. It was their responsibility to find the form, complete it correctly, mail it, and do so in a timely fashion. Filling out the paperwork was particularly difficult for people without bank accounts and those with informal work.[80] Rather than helping patients with this process, hospitals regularly sent bills to collections without ever seeking to find out just how poor the patients were. In an article in *Healthcare Financial Management*, Ray Lefton, an executive at one of Temple University's teaching hospitals in a poor neighborhood in Philadelphia, described debt collection as an "information gathering process" hospitals could use to determine whether a patient was eligible for charity-care or not.[81]

For some, the time spent dealing with hospital collection and lawsuits added insult to serious injury. Lesszest George, a working single mother, cared for her 19-year-old son during and after his hospitalization in the Illinois Masonic Hospital in Chicago after he was shot in 2004. Her son was no longer covered by her insurance after his high school graduation. He was working part-time while he continued his studies, but he had no insurance of his own. When the hospital sent her a bill for $52,000, Lesszest applied for assistance from a Victims' Assistance Fund, but her application was denied. Then, the hospital sued her. So after sleepless nights at her son's bedside, she faced the prospect of massive debts and court dates.[82]

Even when patients and their families thought they were protected by insurance, many found themselves in a Kafkaesque nightmare. After 17-year-old Jolynda Contee was discharged from the Shock Trauma Center in Baltimore, Maryland, in 1993 following serious injuries sustained in an auto accident, her family received a bill for $61,953. Her parents, Albert and Velma Contee, worked for minimum wage at a dry cleaner and had no hope of paying the bill. Their savings, all of $2,000, had been quickly wiped out by all the expenses that came from caring for an injured child. Albert did not worry about the bill at first. After all, he was not rich, but he did have health insurance. But then Albert found out that his insurance would not cover his daughter's medical bills. It was not its responsibility, the company said, because Jolynda was not part of their household since she had been living with a relative, not in her parent's home.

This was a stunning blow, but Albert thought of another possible solution. If his teenage daughter was not to be considered part of his household but had no money of her own, could she obtain assistance from the state? The hospital told him this was not possible because his daughter was not legally emancipated and could not apply on her own. When Albert submitted an application for hospital financial assistance, the hospital denied that, too.

The Contees wanted to pay their bill but had no options. The hospital showed no mercy. It faced $394 million in uncompensated care that year, up from $188 million just 5 years earlier, and sought to recoup some of its losses through aggressive collection. So the Contees joined dozens of former Shock Trauma patients who found themselves being sued by the very hospital whose doctors, weeks earlier, had promised to do everything they could to keep their lives intact.[83]

What was disappearing was the sense that settling unpaid medical debts should involve more than collecting dollars and cents. When debts had involved personal obligations between a doctor and patient, it was understood that there was more than money at stake. The need to maintain an ongoing relationship based on trust and care had remained part of the calculus. But once a debt was just a number on a spreadsheet, sent out to a third party for collection, its moral valence changed. Anthropologist David Graeber's explanation of what happens when a personal obligation becomes an impersonal debt is worth quoting at length, because it explains much of what happened with medical debt:

> A debt is an obligation to pay a certain sum of money. As a result, a debt, unlike any other form of obligation, can be precisely quantified. This allows debts to become simple, cold, and impersonal—which, in turn, allows them to be transferable. If one owes a favor, or one's life, to another human being—it is owed to that person specifically. But if one owes forty thousand dollars at 12 percent interest, it doesn't really matter who the creditor is; neither does either of the two parties have to think much about what the other party needs, wants, is capable of doing—as they certainly would if what was owed was a favor, or respect, or gratitude. One does not need to calculate the human effects; one need only calculate principal, balances, penalties, and rates of interest. If you end up having to abandon your home and wander in other provinces, if your daughter

ends up in a mining camp working as a prostitute, well, that's unfortunate, but incidental to the creditor. Money is money, and a deal's a deal. From this perspective, the crucial factor . . . is money's capacity to turn morality into a matter of personal arithmetic—and by doing so, to justify things that would otherwise seem outrageous or obscene.[84]

In this world of medical, financial, and legal peril, people such as Ms. Wilson were made to toil in a hospital laundry to repay medical debts. They were not alone. Hospitals throughout the country started touting their own programs to put debtors to work in their hospitals. In 1998, executives at Franklin Memorial Hospital in Farmington, Maine, began encouraging patients as well as their friends and family members to work in the hospital to help pay off debts. A 59-year-old woman who had her gallbladder removed faced $4,000 she could not hope to pay. So instead she did clerical work at the hospital for 20 hours each week for 4 months. A 24-year-old carpenter who had undergone wrist surgery to recover his livelihood was trying to spend some of his earnings from his regular job to pay part of his bill in installments; he could not afford the entire $2,400. So every weekend he went into the emergency room, where he made beds and ran blood samples to the lab. Franklin Memorial was proud of this program, touting it as a "Contract for Care" to *Healthcare PR and Marketing News*, an industry journal.[85]

Here is the rub, though. To qualify for the program, a patient's income had to fall below the federal poverty level. These were, by definition, poor patients who were not being given charity-care. The hospital executives claimed they often used up the $500,000 they allocated for charity-care each year, so they were looking for another option for these patients. Instead of setting aside more funds to ensure free or discounted care for low-income patients, the hospital touted the opportunity it afforded them to perform long hours of menial work for the hospital. A Franklin Memorial executive called its Contract for Care a "marketing dream" because it instilled so much "self-esteem" in the patients it had given the opportunity to enter into debt peonage.[86] The idea of putting patients to work to pay for their care had been revived, but now the work carried with it an implicit threat. If they did not toil, patients faced the specter of financial ruin.

PART II

*The Players: Collectors, Hospitals,
Politicians, and Patients*

CHAPTER 3

Trading in Misery

We know that poverty is unpleasant. . . . But don't expect us to do anything about it. . . . The present state of affairs suits us, and we are not going to take the risk of setting you free. . . . So, dear brothers, since evidently you must sweat to pay for our trips to Italy, sweat and be damned to you.

— George Orwell, *Down and Out in Paris and London*

The people who run debt collection firms can be coy. Trade journals and company websites offer all sorts of euphemisms for debt collection, such as "receivables management" or "revenue cycle management." Publicity materials and job recruitment videos foreground companies' commitment to "Christian values," or wellness, or the potential for advancement, or the hours spent volunteering. Mentions of health care debt collection are clothed in comforting language about working with people to come to mutually agreeable solutions.[1] They acknowledge that some people complain about harassing calls, but not to worry: "On an annual basis, debt-buying industry representatives engage in billions of consumer contacts," so the complaints represent a small share of their interactions.[2]

The money debt collectors extract from patients is not framed as a drain on people's financial security but, rather, as a boon to hospital bottom lines and local economies. Collection agencies "employ thousands of U.S. taxpayers nationwide and operate in all 50 states."[3] Buyers of hospital debt argue that hospitals benefit from the revenues secured by selling receivables. An industry association of third-party collection agencies, ACA International, commissioned a survey which found that "the collection industry returned $44.6 billion to creditors in 2010." This figure includes all kinds of debt, although health care–related debt accounted for 52.6 percent, or $23.5 billion.[4]

Debt collection executives do not usually solicit press attention. Yet some of the most brash in the business disclaim any squeamishness about making money off debt. As one hard-nosed investor explained to journalist Jake Halpern, "People make mistakes, but [the debt collector] didn't put them in debt, they were just trying to collect. If the pitcher makes a bad pitch and the batter hits a home run, the batter isn't in the wrong, he's just doing his job."[5]

This was an unusually frank admission. Normally, only by reading marketing materials aimed not at the general public but at hospital chief financial officers (CFOs) seeking to assign or sell debt, or to banks with capital to finance their work, do you realize the nature of the work. Here the companies impress upon the reader the size of the market and the efficiency of collection. They promise to deliver CFOs more of their uncollected debt, and to do it quickly.

The medical debt collection industry includes a few different kinds of businesses. In federal law, the term "debt collectors" is taken to include collection agencies, debt buyers, and collection law firms (often hired by other companies and by originating creditors to pursue debts through litigation). Indeed, many companies include elements of all three subtypes. It is not uncommon for an agency to own some debt outright, receive other debt on contingency, and employ lawyers to pursue debtors in court.[6]

As of 2022, there were roughly 6,300 debt collection firms in the United States. The number was on the decline, falling from roughly 10,000 in 2012, as buyouts created larger companies and the industry became more concentrated.[7] A survey of these firms conducted in 2015 by the Consumer Financial Protection Bureau (CFPB) demonstrated that most of them were small; 75 percent had fewer than 20 employees. Revenues in the industry were concentrated in larger firms; the 25 percent of firms with more than 20 employees accounted for 86 percent of industry revenue.[8]

Collecting medical debt is a huge portion of the work of these firms, and the collection tactics for medical debt are particularly aggressive. Most firms in the 2015 CFPB survey collected medical debt, and for 29 percent of firms, medical collection drove the majority of revenue. Of those companies, 88 percent sued debtors and 100 percent reported delinquent debt to credit bureaus. These firms were far more likely to resort to this measure than firms that collected primarily credit card or student loan debt, despite the fact that the balances owed by people with medical debts were on average much smaller than other kinds of debt; medical debt balances were typically below $1,000.[9]

For the rank-and-file agents, debt collection is not particularly remunerative or enjoyable work. In 2015, entry-level agents earned approximately $11 per hour, below the national median hourly wage of roughly $13 per hour. Most collection agents could earn incentives; one typical package stipulated that after meeting a certain threshold, collectors could earn 25 percent of the contingency fee. Their workdays are spent mostly making calls. Typically, a collector is responsible for roughly 2,000 accounts at a time, and they might call a debtor two or three times each week until the account is settled. To facilitate the sheer volume of calls, many firms pay for predictive dialers, which are automated systems that use algorithms to predict an agent's availability and place the next phone call before they have finished the previous one. The incessant pace and low pay help explain why larger companies have annual turnover rates between 75 and 100 percent.[10]

Thus, most people employed by debt collection companies are not that different from the people they call. Both typically work long hours at low wages to pay bills. Just as women are more likely to carry medical debt, they are also more likely to work the phones to collect it. In a nationwide survey commissioned by ACA International and published in 2022, women made up 72 percent of collection agents.[11] ACA International heralded this fact on Twitter as a triumph for diversity, but few people make rewarding careers of this labor.

There are, however, industry leaders who have made a fortune from medical debt collection. For some of these empire-builders, medical debt has been their ticket to wealth and prestige. Some of these leaders built their companies from tiny operations into huge corporations. Others bought existing operations to fold into multibillion-dollar enterprises. Still others combined ambitions in business and politics by winning public office and then seeking to halt attempts to regulate the industry. The stories of three companies—NCO Financial, RR Resource Recovery, and Capio Partners—demonstrate not only the fortunes that are to be gained in debt collection but also how the rise of this class of intermediaries between doctor and patient has allowed an ethos of impersonal financialization, of profit maximization, to overwhelm older notions of obligation. Once these old bonds were deemed quaint and outdated, aggressive collection tactics could run rampant.

Michael Barrist was chief executive officer (CEO) of NCO Financial Systems, which was, by 1992, a rapidly growing debt collection company based outside Philadelphia. Barrist's company had come a long way since his grandfather, Louis Barrist, had founded it in 1926. Back then, debt collection involved agents standing outside tenements, shouting into megaphones for the debtor to come out and pay his department-store bill or overdue rent.[12]

Michael Barrist bought the family firm from his mother in 1986, 2 years after graduating from Drexel University with a degree in accounting. His mother had been running the company with three employees out of her home garage. The company had only 60 clients and an annual revenue of $40,000. Michael paid $25,000 for the firm and quickly moved it out of the garage to a small office in Rosemont, a suburb of Philadelphia.

Determined to make something more of the tiny operation, Barrist hired Charles Piola, a former high school teacher who had become a leading area sales representative for debt collection services. Piola was, according to *Inc.* magazine, the "king of cold calls." Once at NCO, he made unannounced visits to office buildings, where he tried to convince executives to hire the firm to collect their debts. Driving a Mercedes and dressed in a double-breasted, pinstriped suit, a cashmere topcoat, and freshly shined shoes, and carrying an expensive leather briefcase, he ambled into law offices, ophthalmology practices, insurance companies, banks, and almost any other business acting as if he belonged until he found someone who looked like they controlled the books, and then he would strike up a conversation. He attributed his success to his friendliness and his indifference to rejection.[13] So devoted was Piola to this identity that when he eventually left the company, he became a motivational speaker, attempting to rouse business audiences with such themes as "Christ Was a Cold Call Salesman."[14]

For his part, Barrist aimed to use software to partially automate the process of sending letters and making calls. Today, these "collection management systems"—software platforms that for a monthly subscription fee help collectors track calls, payments, and conversations with debtors—are standard throughout the industry.[15] But at the time, they were rare, and due in part to this automation, NCO could offer lower contingency fees than the competition. The company took as little as 11 percent of the debt collected, whereas other agencies demanded at least 20 percent.[16] With this combination of shoe-leather charm, cutting-edge software, and cut-rate offers, NCO was able to rapidly expand its client list.

And while NCO's clients were many and varied, including the Philadelphia 76ers, AT&T, and Mellon Bank, medical debt was their major focus. After an economic recession in the early 1990s, Barrist's clientele grew even faster. "A lot of doctors in the past year have decided to use collectors for the first time because they have to do it," he told the *Philadelphia Inquirer* in 1992.[17] In the company's first few years, Piola said he cold-called hundreds of doctors' offices, hospitals, and medical clinics.[18] By 1991, the company mailed out 120,000 computer-generated collection letters every month for its 1,700 clients, of which 70 percent were medical.[19]

Barrist and Piola admitted that medical debt collection involved difficult conversations. Barrist lamented that "most people want to pay their bills, they just don't have the money."[20] But their business model proved a smashing success. Part of his promise was that he could relieve doctors of the grubby work of pursuing overdue bills. As Piola explained:

> [Companines] hate chasing after delinquent accounts. Professional people, especially doctors, lawyers and accountants, find it undignified to hound patients and clients who refuse to pay bills. That's not their business. But it was *our* business, and over time we became very adept at it.[21]

Through aggressive collection tactics and buyouts of rival collection firms, the company grew so large that it became known as "the Wal-Mart of debt collection."[22] How did it go about collecting debts? A reporter for *Inc.* magazine got a sense of it as he followed Piola through Wills Eye Hospital in Philadelphia, where the salesman was in his element, striking up conversations and handing his business card to any administrator he could find. Piola happened across the new manager of an ocular oncology practice, who told him about her frustration collecting bills. Piola described how NCO would collect from one of her delinquent patients: "After four or five months in our system he's going to get 45 or 50 attempts. We'll send letters. We'll do skip tracing [i.e., track down debtors who change addresses]. We'll get a neighbor to tell us where he works and go after him there." Impressed, the manager offered him a contract on the spot.[23]

Barrist took the firm public in 1996. In its initial public offering, the firm was valued at $30 million. Barrist's star and his net worth continued to rise alongside the rapid rise in consumer debt. Shares of NCO nearly tripled in value in the company's first 6 months as a publicly traded company. Revenues rose from $30 million in 1996 to more than $100 million in 1998; during this period, NCO acquired 11 companies.

The local papers wrote of Barrist's rise with wonder, even pride, befitting a local boy made good, with nary a word about the maladies and financial hardships that made his fortune possible. "I never dreamed in a million years that NCO would be what it has become in size," he told a reporter for the *Philadelphia Inquirer*.[24] But he was nowhere near satisfied. In an interview for the *Philadelphia Business Journal*, Barrist attributed his success to his work ethic, estimating he worked at least 65 hours each week. In 1998, his compensation totaled $1.3 million.[25] NCO was the fastest-growing debt collection company in the country and, the next year, after another round of acquisitions, it was the largest.[26] By August 2001, NCO had 8,400 employees and was worth $529 million.[27]

Medical debt collection was a large part of NCO's work. These were, in the words of Albert Zezulinski, Executive Vice President of Global Portfolio Operations at NCO, "fresh and fertile markets."[28] The company bought debt from ambulance companies and hospitals as well as from groups of emergency physicians, radiologists, and anesthesiologists. In 2007, the company devoted 2,000 of its 9,000 collectors to medical debt.[29] An NCO subsidiary called Transworld Systems even signed an agreement with the American Medical Association (AMA) to become the preferred provider of debt collection services to the organization's membership. The AMA leadership immediately took to promoting Transworld's services; Robert Musacchio, a senior vice president, said, "Transworld's easy online system can help busy physicians manage their receivables quickly allowing them to focus on what they do best—care for patients."[30]

After buying yet more companies and following unforeseen delays in client contracts, NCO's share price fell in 2000. To appease shareholders wary of continued buyouts while satiating his own appetite for more growth, Barrist announced the formation of a separate debt-purchasing business called NCO Portfolio Management. This company focused on debt buying and used the NCO Group's existing infrastructure to collect the debts.[31]

During the early 2000s, Barrist was enthusiastic about purchasing medical debt, particularly because "the markets are less developed and there's less competition" than in other areas of consumer debt.[32] On an earnings call, he told analysts that he expected hospitals to begin selling large volumes of debt for two reasons. First, debt purchasers were trying to find new investments, "so they're going to start waving larger amounts under these hospitals' noses." Second, hospitals facing budgetary woes "are going to have to face up to the fact that they need alternate means to generate cash in the door." His "challenge," he explained, was "getting a hospital client to crack and basically let us buy [their debt]."[33]

As detailed in Chapter 2, by the mid-2000s medical debt buying had gone mainstream. More hospital CFOs turned to selling both bad debt and accounts that had not yet even gone into default. Joel Lewis, an executive at a holding company for Medclr, an established debt buyer that partnered with NCO on debt purchases, explained, "The trend of selling bad debt in the general consumer debt area proved successful and is now being applied to the medical universe."[34] The business was also becoming more predictable due to "forward-flow deals" in which hospitals and physician groups agreed to sell the buyer a certain amount of debt each month.[35]

For a time, the debt buying model proved successful, and Barrist continued to shine as a titan of business. In 2006, he worked with One Equity Partners, the private equity unit of the investment bank J. P. Morgan Chase, to buy out NCO for $1.26 billion.[36] In 2011, Drexel University, Barrist's alma mater, named him to its alumni hall of fame.[37]

But Barrist was eventually a victim of his own success. In part because medical debt collection had become so popular, its profitability soon abated. Cost-cutting and automation, the kinds of disruptions that Barrist had long championed, pushed down contingent fees (the percentage of collected debts that went to the collection agency) from as high as 40 percent during the 1980s to as low as 10 percent by the 2010s. Meanwhile, hospitals were becoming more effective at collecting on their own from people with the means to pay before they went into default, so recovery rates for third-party debt collectors fell, from 25 percent in the early 1980s to 10 percent three decades later.[38] Barrist attempted to increase profitability by using call centers in low-wage locations such as India, the Philippines, Central America, and the Caribbean, but this cost cutting could only go so far.[39]

Finding more debt to buy was another problem for Barrist. Seeking out medical accounts to service was more challenging than buying from huge credit card companies, as thousands of hospitals made their own individual decisions about whether and where to sell debt. Health care debts were also smaller on average than credit card debts, so the per-dollar cost of collecting was often higher. When large corporations entered the market for medical debt in the mid-2000s, they offered hospitals higher prices than existing buyers, pushing the price of debt higher. When these new entrants to the market found debts more difficult to buy in large quantities and less profitable than expected, some pulled out. Encore Capital stopped buying and collecting medical debt in 2007. Portfolio Recovery closed its health care division in 2009, and in 2010, Asset Acceptance sold its remaining medical debt to Capio Partners. In 2010, NCO Group also stopped buying medical debt, although it continued to collect on a contingency basis.[40]

In 2011, after a period of losses, NCO's board fired Barrist as CEO. He did receive a $3.4 million severance payment and was allowed to remain chairman of the board. The board replaced him with Ronald Rittenmeyer, a longtime executive at companies ranging from Frito-Lay, Inc. to AIG and for-profit hospital operator Tenet Healthcare.[41] J. P. Morgan then combined NCO Financial Systems with other debt collection firms to form a holding company called Expert Global Solutions. This was, at the time, the largest debt collector in the world, with 42,000 workers at 120 call centers worldwide.

In addition to its dominant position in the world of debt collection, NCO and its successor, Expert Global, became well-known for illegal collection tactics. In 2004, NCO paid a $1.5 million fine to the Federal Trade Commission (FTC)—at the time, the largest fine it had ever levied—for failing to file timely records to clear debts from the credit reports of debtors who had paid what they owed. In 2012, after a prolonged investigation, NCO agreed to pay $1 million in a settlement involving 19 states to refund customers who had been harassed into paying debts they did not actually owe.[42] The next year, Expert Global set a new record for an FTC fine when it paid $3.2 million, this time for violating the Fair Debt Collections Practices Act. The FTC complaint laid out the violations in detail. Collectors failed to verify that the people they contacted were the actual debtors, even after the people contacted insisted that the debts were not theirs. Collectors called multiple times per day, or at the debtors' place of employment, or after being asked to stop, with what the FTC called an "intent to annoy, harass, or abuse."[43]

Barrist was not done with the industry that had made him rich. Soon after leaving NCO in 2012, he announced plans to lead a new venture, Radius Global Solutions. With this company, Barrist pledged "to not just reenter the industry but to transform it" with novel uses of communications technology to reach debtors.[44] Although never as large as his other venture, it did return him to the work of collecting medical debt.

Barrist had been a trailblazer in medical debt collection, and other companies followed his lead. Particularly after credit card debt fell in the wake of the 2008 financial crisis, medical debt emerged as a crucial source of revenue for collection agencies. Even if debt buying and debt collection on contingency both proved less profitable than evangelists such as Barrist had claimed in the mid-2000s, they were still big business, particularly as other forms of consumer debt fell. The FTC surveyed the nine largest debt buyers in the United States in 2013, which reported owning more than 21 million medical accounts, with an average face value of $345.[45] Four years later, medical debt was the most common reason Americans were contacted by debt collectors.[46] Medical debt collection had entered the mainstream and piqued the interest of some of the world's richest people.

One of those people would soon buy out Barrist's former company. In 2014, the medical debt portion of Expert Global Solutions was placed under the aegis of a subsidiary called Transworld Systems Inc. (TSI) and sold to a private equity firm called Platinum Equity.[47] This firm was headquartered in Beverly Hills, California, and owned by billionaire Tom Gores. According to *Forbes* Magazine, as of July 2022, Gores was the 424th wealthiest person in the world, just behind Twitter founder Jack Dorsey and *Star Wars* creator

George Lucas. Gores was best known as owner of the National Basketball Association's Detroit Pistons and as a philanthropist.[48] He was a member of the board of directors of the UCLA Medical Center as well as a donor to Children's Hospital Los Angeles and to various causes in Detroit and Flint, Michigan, where he had grown up.[49] He was a pillar in the civic life of two great American cities.

Gores was also the owner of a debt collection machine, a network of call centers and legal teams and software designed to chase down patients who owed medical bills. Under his stewardship, TSI was not nearly as charitable as his public image would suggest. In 2017, the CFPB fined the company $2.5 million for illegally suing people for student debt. The company hired a network of law firms to file and prosecute collection lawsuits, but consumers were sued for debt that companies either could not prove was owed or had passed the statute of limitations. According to the CFPB, the affidavits filed by these law firms falsely claimed personal knowledge of account records.[50]

In medical debt, TSI did not have a better reputation. By 2017, it was the company with the most complaints related to medical debt in the CFPB's database.[51] One person in Georgia claimed that TSI had called a friend to find him (which is allowed) but during that call had said it was in regard to a medical debt that he owed (which is not allowed).[52] A resident of Illinois complained that a negative action had been filed on his credit report by TSI for a medical debt that he had never heard of and was sure he did not owe. He said he had tried to call TSI numerous times to settle the matter, but he could never get anyone on the other end of the line.[53] Another person in Missouri claimed that TSI called his work cell phone so often, and despite his pleas to contact him at home instead, that his supervisor became annoyed and passed him over for a pay raise.[54]

The 2010s were an era of massive private equity inroads into health care billing and collection. As hospitals struggled to find the staff to collect on growing unpaid patient bills while complying with new regulations, private equity–owned firms promised a "one-stop shop" where hospitals could outsource the work of "revenue cycle management" in its entirety. These companies promised to handle the initial work of billing, and not just collection on delinquent accounts.[55] Such companies used information technology alongside dogged collection tactics to pursue medical debt. The CFPB found that these kinds of companies were particularly quick to report debts to credit reporting agencies when they met any delays in collecting payments.[56]

There were other medical collection executives in high places. In 2010, 38-year-old Tom Reed ran as a Republican for the United States House of

Representatives in New York's 29th Congressional District, a rural region in the state's western reaches. As Mayor of Corning, a city with a population of 11,000, Reed often called himself a "country lawyer." A portly man with a mild manner, a soft voice, and conservative politics, Reed portrayed himself as a break from the past after taking the seat of former Democratic Representative Eric Massa, who resigned from Congress after being accused of sexual harassment by his own staffers.

But despite his man-of-the-people image, Reed made his living in medical debt collection and litigation. His law firm's business came in large part from suing his own constituents for unpaid debts on behalf of Corning Hospital and its parent health system, Guthrie.[57] That did not keep Reed from winning the election, defeating Matt Zeller, a former Central Intelligence Agency analyst and veteran of the war in Afghanistan.

Critiques of Reed's business surfaced in a 2014 article in *The Buffalo News*, which reported that Reed's law firm continued to file lawsuits even after he took office. The controversy surrounding this revelation centered mostly on the fact that House ethics rules forbade lawmakers from practicing law or allowing their names to be used by law firms.[58] Reed's team gave varied rationalizations for the violation. His attorney told a reporter that members of the office staff may have used old stationery. Reed himself gave the rather lame excuse that he had not changed the name of the firm because he had no name to change it to.[59] Even after finally removing his name from the firm, his family continued to benefit from its work. Ownership was transferred in part to his wife, Jean, and his brother John. The name of the law office was changed to RR Resource Recovery, and the congressman continued to claim income from the company's operations on House ethics disclosures.[60]

Only later did the public focus change from the issue of House rules to the fact that as a mayor and congressman, Reed had profited off the financial misery and suffering of his own constituents. One such constituent, Michael Enslow, complained that RR Resource Recovery refused to remove a medical debt from his credit report long after he repaid it. He complained that the knock on his credit prevented him from being preapproved for a mortgage. Other people filed complaints with the FTC and the CFPB against the firm Reed founded, claiming negative actions taken on their credit reports for bills for care they had never received.

A complainant from Hallstead, Pennsylvania, said that after he heard from his credit union that his credit score had dropped, he looked at his credit report. There he found that RR Resource Recovery had filed a negative action for a past-due medical bill for $13 from an appointment 2 years earlier. When he asked why he had never been notified by the collection agency prior to this action on his credit report, the collector told him it was company policy to inform credit bureaus without contacting debtors for any bills of less than $20. When he asked how he could be expected to know to pay the bill, the collector said that was his problem, then asked how he would like to pay.[61] At a town hall meeting, a local consumer rights attorney confronted Congressman Reed, claiming RR Resource Recovery sued uninsured patients on behalf of local hospitals.[62]

Reed's politics aligned closely with his financial interests. He was, unsurprisingly, a vocal critic of the "unelected, independent bureaucrats" at the CFPB. He voted for a bill that would weaken the agency's power to regulate "unfair, deceptive and abusive practices."[63] He also appeared as a guest on cable television programs to argue for the repeal of the Affordable Care Act, which would have thrown millions of Americans off of Medicaid rolls and spurred increased medical debts. He was a prolific fundraiser and a member of the powerful House Ways and Means Committee, which held authority over writing taxes. In early 2022, he openly contemplated a run for governor of New York. But when a lobbyist named Nicolette Davis stepped forward to accuse Reed of unclipping her bra and putting his hand on her thigh in a Minneapolis bar 5 years earlier, he resigned from Congress to join a lobbying firm.[64]

Not all debt collectors face such personal and professional ruin. Capio, founded in 2008 by Jim Richards and Mark Detrick, is one of the nation's largest debt purchasers. The company claims it has purchased portfolios from more than 750 hospitals, as well as physician groups, with a face value of $32 billion. In exchange for this portfolio of debt, it has paid health care providers more than $250 million. Capio has collected on the debts of 20 million patients "to create practical and personalized solutions to help them pay their fair share of medical expenses."[65]

The company's founders are old hands in medical debt collection. Richards has a gravelly voice that brims with confidence, with the assured sense that he has seen it all. And, in the world of medical debt, he had. Prior to Capio, Richards spent decades as an executive at Medaphis Services Corp., Attention, and West Asset Management. At each company, Richards had grown the medical debt collection business, securing ever larger contracts with health care providers. In 2008, Richards and his partners founded Capio because they believed they had amassed the expertise and experience to become the premier buyer of medical debt:

We saw about 25 players in the healthcare debt-buying business. . . . We didn't think any of them were quite as qualified as us. They had little collection agencies that didn't know debt buying, and big debt buyers that didn't know health care, and we saw an opportunity to own that space.[66]

Capio Partners' collection tactics quickly became a subject of critical attention. In 2011, the *Atlanta Journal-Constitution* reported that in 2 years, Capio had been sued in federal court 15 times for alleged violations of the Fair Debt Collection Practices Act. These suits claimed that the company had tried to collect on bills previously discharged in bankruptcy, had reported bills to credit bureaus beyond the statute of limitations, and had harassed debtors over the phone.

In one such complaint, Sherry Bates of Conroe, Texas, claimed that after she disputed the validity of her bill, the agent told her to pay it anyway, even if she did not owe the money. When Bates refused, Capio reported the debt to a credit bureau, even though the time limit for reporting the debt had passed, then called her so often that she changed her phone number. Bates eventually settled her case.[67]

Five years later, Capio was again in the news. The *St. Louis Post-Dispatch* chronicled more than 1,000 lawsuits filed against area residents over 16 months for care at local emergency rooms run by SSM Health, a not-for-profit health system with a self-professed "special concern for people who are poor and vulnerable." Among the patients sued for hospital bills—at a Catholic hospital—was a local priest.

But control of the debt had moved far from its faith-based, nonprofit roots. Physician staffing of most of SSM's emergency departments had been outsourced to a for-profit company called Schumacher Clinical Partners, which had been purchased by the private equity firm Onex Partners in 2015. Schumacher Clinical Partners sold its bad debt to Capio Partners, which then hired CP Medical LLC, another legal firm specializing in collection and based in Las Vegas, Nevada. When the *Post-Dispatch* asked SSM's executives about the lawsuits, they claimed they had no idea their patients were being taken to court.

The hospital executives' plea of ignorance was not entirely credible. Any legal action against patients required the approval of the director of the hospital's patient service center. Even with this required communication, SSM and Schumacher did little to ensure that charity-care was handled collaboratively. Schumacher's CFO admitted that it did not automatically forgive the debts of patients who were given charity-care by the hospital.

When Capio did take debtors to court, it was almost always successful. The defendants were represented by lawyers in only 17 of the 1,078 cases reviewed by the *Post-Dispatch*. "They're a default judgment machine," said Robert Swearingen, an attorney with Legal Services of Eastern Missouri who represented some of the defendants.[68] After winning the cases, the collection lawyers aimed to recoup their debts by garnishing wages and seizing bank accounts.

Capio's leaders are not marginal figures in the industry. Richards was president of the board of ACA International and was awarded the inaugural "Integrity Award" from the Receivables Management Association. In extolling his partner upon receiving this honor, Detrick explained, "Our approach to serving patients is to treat each person as an individual and provide them with options to resolve their healthcare expense obligations."[69]

In a 2016 interview, recorded just a month before the *St. Louis Post-Dispatch* exposé went to press, Richards explained his aim was to change the perception of the industry, which had grown so negative as to rouse unwelcome attention from legislators and regulators. He had even founded an Institute for Collection Leadership, which would pool the "time, talent and treasure" of leading third-party collectors, debt buyers, and law firms to advance the claim that they were being unfairly maligned. His goal was to raise millions of dollars to hire lobbyists to defend the industry.

Richards offered some lines of argument in defense of his work: "When [policymakers] hear that there are 100,000 complaints, that sounds like a lot, until you look at [the fact that] there are billions of calls and letters sent out." And in any case, he argued, debt collection had evolved:

> The industry has changed. We used to just call up, ask for the balance in full, potentially threaten something. . . . Today we are all about customer-centric issues. We are more caring, we are more understanding, we are more financial counselors. . . . We are here to get stuff off of the customer's plate and help them with their credit."[70]

Thus, even as his company was the target of investigative journalists and consumer complaints, Richards worked to shape the public image so that these critiques would not lead to policy changes harmful to the bottom line. He hoped that health care debt buying would grow. By repairing the perception of the industry, he aimed to convince more hospitals to sell debt. In 2016, he said that "even today . . . only 8 or 9 percent of hospital decision makers have sold debt, and we are working on that 15–16 percent tipping point number to where everyone is doing it." He admitted he was spending lots of money on marketing, trying to convince hospitals that they could "get that last penny out of the receivable for them," after other efforts at collection had failed.[71]

After four decades in the industry, Richards' ambition has only grown. Capio's website advises potential clients that it is looking for "high volume engagements."[72] Seeking to overcome the well-trod difficulty of managing a large debt-buying company by amassing relatively small purchases from many different hospitals, Capio seeks a minimum of $50 million in annual uncollectible receivables with each contract.

The company website promises to conduct business "with the highest degree of professionalism and respect for clients and their patients."[73] In a 2022 interview, CEO Mark Detrick explained that the company had never charged interest or fees (common in the industry) and, after the 2016 *Post-Dispatch* article, had stopped suing patients. It also does not resell debt.[74] When asked about the consumer complaints to the CFPB, Detrick argued that most of them "reflect consumer confusion, not poor treatment"; these are, he contended, legitimate debts that they patients not recognize or did not realize had not been paid by their insurers. Detrick admitted that despite their efforts to verify debts and treat debtors with respect, "our agents are human," and "sometimes we do make mistakes." He argued that training and quality review of calls would ensure that the interactions with debtors "meet our standards for customer experience."[75] Capio also claimed that it had forgiven $356 million in patient debt since 2008, though this amounts to only 1.1 percent of the face value of its debt.

Detrick and Richards remain vocal defenders of the debt-buying industry, speaking on podcasts and before university symposia and opposing state-level attempts to ban the purchase of medical debt. They also continue to sell their services to hospitals around the country. On its website, Capio advised hospitals that selling debt was a powerful motivation for repayment, as it "creates an expectation of payment within their patient base and enhances performance."[76] But why would selling debt improve repayment if not for fear of debt buyers and their tactics? This fear, it turns out, is merited, and not only when medical debt is held by a third party. Hospitals themselves have been some of the most aggressive collectors of their patients' debts. The most infamous case is the subject of the next chapter.

CHAPTER 4

Out of the Shadows

Medical Debt Collection in the Press and in
Political Debate

If someone told me this story, I would've told them they were lying. I had no idea someone
would go after someone in such a vicious way. They made my life a living nightmare.
—Joseph Jackson, as cited in *Uncharitable Care: Yale New Haven's Charity Care*
and Collections Practices

By 2003, a majority of hospitals reported suing patients in civil courts,
aiming to garnish wages or seize assets for unpaid debts.[1] This practice had gone under the radar of public attention until the aggressive debt
collection of Yale New Haven Hospital (YNHH), the major teaching hospital of Yale University and the largest hospital in Connecticut, became
national news, when the hospital's lawsuits against patients were covered
in a series of exposés in the *Wall Street Journal*. But uncovering this practice, and bringing it to public attention, was actually a more grassroots
process, one that involved local groups and dogged researchers. Medical
debt collection would become an issue of national political importance in
the mid-2000s through the efforts of strange bedfellows: union organizers
and arch-conservative activists, reporters from local alt-weeklies and national newspapers, a mild-mannered Pennsylvania congressman, and a
Mississippi trial attorney destined for federal prison.

It was not a national daily, but a now-defunct alt-weekly, *The New
Haven Advocate*, that first brought YNHH's practice of suing patients to

light. One former editor of the paper remembered it as "a combination of arts coverage and progressive politics" that was, for decades, "an absolute must-read—not only among the heads, freaks and geeks and other counter-culturalists who loitered on the Green (smoking the green), but in the political and business communities, too."[2] An article in the May 31, 2001, issue, "Predator on the Hill," was written by reporter and editor Paul Bass, a bearded, vegan, longtime New Haven resident who was locally well-known as a progressive muckraker (Figures 4.1a and 4.1b). In it, Bass highlighted the hospital's practice of foreclosing on the homes of patients, some of whom worked low-paying jobs at the hospital, over unpaid debts. But hospital executive Marna Borgstrom insisted YNHH was in

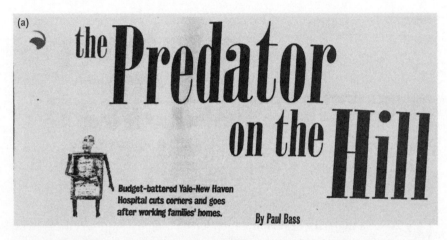

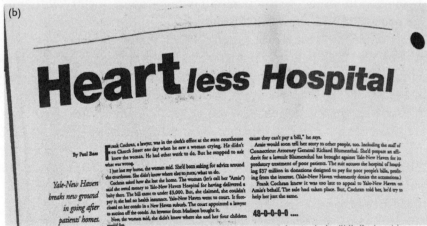

Figure 4.1: Headlines by Paul Bass in *The New Haven Advocate* on lawsuits against patients by Yale New Haven Hospital.
Source: Paul Bass, *The New Haven Advocate*, May 31, 2001 (top), and April 17, 2003 (bottom).

the right, arguing that these lawsuits were "the only way we are going to be able to provide free care" to the poor. Claiming that the hospital only sued patients with the ability to pay, she blamed debtors for their lax spending habits: "I'm always amazed at what people pay for discretionary items."[3]

YNHH's claims would not withstand the scrutiny of another reader of Bass' reporting. Grace Rollins was a recent graduate of Yale and a researcher for a local chapter of the Service Employees International Union (SEIU), which was in the midst of organizing food service workers at YNHH. Alongside community advocates, legal aid groups, and labor organizations, Rollins compiled a report, "Uncharitable Care," on YNHH's collection practices.[4] Released in January 2003, the report recounted the experiences of a number of New Haven residents, many employed by the hospital, who had been sued for delinquent bills. Most of the patients she profiled struggled to get by on low incomes. Some were uninsured, and others had been billed in error. But YNHH collectors were relentless in their pursuit of debts that totaled in the tens (and sometimes hundreds) of thousands of dollars, despite the fact that YNHH was a tax-exempt institution that reported revenues $20 million in excess of expenses in 2001 alone, due in large part to public subsidies intended for the care of the uninsured.

Beyond the personal tales of woe, Rollins highlighted the actors behind the lawsuits. The hospital's two highest paid independent contractors were Tobin & Melien, a collection law firm based in New Haven, and Century Collection Agency, based in neighboring North Haven. In fiscal year 2002, with the aid of these contractors, YNHH filed more than 400 lawsuits against patients in Connecticut courts. When the hospital won—which it did in the vast majority of cases—it took a number of post-judgment actions to collect.

In the YNHH cases, as in most medical debt–related lawsuits, the most common initial post-judgment action was wage garnishment: The court ordered the debtor's employer to deduct a certain amount (in most states, as high as 25 percent) from her weekly take-home earnings. A judge could modify this amount if the patient pled hardship, but that extended the term of repayment, particularly as interest accrued.[5] The most common reason courts resort to wage garnishment is to collect child support payments, but for millions of Americans, wages are garnished for debts such as student loans and medical bills.[6]

For some debt collectors, garnishing wages was not enough. If a debtor had savings, YNHH's lawyers would sometimes seek a bank execution: The court ordered a seizure of a debtor's bank account up to the amount of the judgment plus fees for the execution itself. When the debtor had less than the amount of the judgment in savings, the entire account could be taken.[7]

Some state legislators, including lawmakers in Connecticut, have proposed laws to exempt some portion of savings from bank execution, but large debt collection firms have lobbied hard against these protections.[8]

If these measures proved insufficient to the hospital's debt collectors, they proceeded to seek a property lien. The word *lien*, a mid-sixteenth-century French term, is derived from the Latin word *ligare*, "to bind." This notion of a bind is the most straightforward way to understand a lien, which gives the creditor a legal right to a debtor's assets to secure payment of a debt. In YNHH's lawsuits against patients, the liens they sought were on patients' homes. Whereas other local hospitals rarely sought liens against patients, YNHH placed them with great alacrity. Between 1994 and 2003, Yale School of Medicine and YNHH placed a medical lien on 7.5 percent of owner-occupied homes in New Haven, a city in which the median income was less than $30,000.[9] The debt need not be large for a creditor to seek a property lien; YNHH placed liens for judgments of less than $1,000. But this act significantly raised the stakes for patients in debt. For a debtor, having a lien on a home limited their ability to sell or refinance their home because their property was, in essence, no longer theirs to decide how to manage. The lien was also reported to credit agencies, which in turn affected debtors' ability to buy or rent a home or, in some cases, even find a job.

Most concerning for the patient, the lien opened the legal path toward foreclosure. After obtaining a lien, if the patient proved unable to settle their debt, YNHH could proceed with another lawsuit to foreclose on the patient's home. Once the hospital won this lawsuit and dispossessed the patient of their home, the hospital would sell the house at auction and use the proceeds to settle the debt. As Rollins noted in her report, patients did have one last refuge at this stage. In order to protect their homes from foreclosure, patients could, and often did, file for bankruptcy[10] because doing so leads a court to issue an automatic stay, preventing creditors from enforcing liens or collecting what they are owed while the court decides how to settle the debts. However, bankruptcy limited patients' access to credit and provided only temporary relief from collectors. Although old debts were settled in the bankruptcy process, the home was not always saved, and patients were likely to incur new debts (including medical debts) all too soon.[11] But for the desperate patients, declaring bankruptcy kept the hospital from seizing their homes, at least for a time.

Rollins' report attracted the attention of Lucette Lagnado, a health care reporter for the *Wall Street Journal*. In early 2003, Rollins arranged for Lagnado to interview Quinton White, an older man whose court records Rollins had come across in her research.[12] White, who was subsequently featured in the first of Lagnado's series of stories on YNHH's aggressive debt collection practices, was a 77-year-old retired man who had worked at a dry cleaner for much of his life. He owed $40,000 to YNHH for two admissions that his wife, Jeanette, had there in 1982. The interest on the debt had been growing at 10 percent for 20 years, alongside legal fees, court costs, and late charges. In 1983, YNHH's lawyers had placed a lien on the Whites' home. They did not stop after Jeanette died of cancer in 1993. In 1996, the hospital's lawyers seized Quinton's bank account—despite the fact that he had steadily repaid Yale $16,000 in installments, close to the amount he originally owed, in a valiant attempt to make good on his debts, even as he struggled with chronic kidney disease that left him dependent on dialysis three times a week. He dreamed of someday going to Paris, which he had only seen in movies, but did not think he would ever be able to afford it.[13]

Readers of the *Wall Street Journal* were incensed by this story. More than 100 people wrote to the paper, expressing outrage and even offering to help White pay off his debt. After hearing of his long-deferred dream to visit Paris, an Air France spokesman offered him two free, round-trip tickets. Others contacted YNHH to complain. E. Richard Brown, founder of the UCLA Center for Health Policy Research and a former health policy adviser to President Bill Clinton, called for federal legislation or an executive order to prevent hospitals that received federal funding from using "draconian" collection practices, including garnishing wages, placing liens on homes, and charging usurious interest rates.[14]

That Quinton White could even be held liable for the debt of his wife was the result of a tangled legal history. Every state law includes a "doctrine of necessaries," which makes parents liable for the support of their children; they must, in other words, provide what is necessary for the health and well-being of their children. In some states, however, this doctrine is also held to make spouses liable for the financial support of one another. This is a relic of seventeenth-century English jurisprudence in which women had no right to own property or assume debts independent of their husbands, so husbands were deemed to have an obligation to pay the necessary expenses of their wives.[15]

This archaic interpretation of the doctrine of necessaries does not exist everywhere: In Georgia, for instance, the spousal doctrine of necessaries has been repealed by the legislature, and in Florida, it has been ruled unconstitutional by the courts.[16] But in states where the spousal doctrine remains, hospitals have used it to sue spouses when patients died in debt. In fact, medical debt is the predominant kind of debt for which the doctrine of necessaries is invoked.[17] Ironically, given the burden the doctrine places on widows and widowers, the very fact that medical care is such a necessary expense is what makes it so easy for hospitals to invoke the doctrine in court.

Being denied charity-care, or facing a negative action on a credit report, or enduring a lawsuit, or a wage garnishment, or a bank execution, or a foreclosure, is traumatizing enough, but it was not the worst fate to befall medical debtors. Once creditors received a court judgment in their favor, they were able to use the court to "discover" where the debtor's assets were located. If a patient failed to appear in court for an oral examination as part of this process of discovery, the creditor could request that the court issue a body attachment directing the sheriff to arrest the debtor, or judges could make the decision to issue the warrant on their own. The debtor was technically being arrested for contempt of court, not the debt, because debtors' prisons were both illegal and, after a 1983 Supreme Court decision, unconstitutional.[18] But the fundamental cause of the arrest was the debt. In 2020, 44 states allowed the arrest of a debtor for failing to appear in court or failing to provide information to creditors after a judgment against them.[19] Medical debtors are frequent targets. In Idaho, for instance, Medical Recovery Services LLC sought and obtained the arrest of more debtors than any other collector in the state between 2010 and 2016. In one case in that state, a judge set bail at more than twice the amount of the debt.[20]

YNHH was one of many hospitals that sought civil arrest warrants if patients did not appear in court; Rollins found that the hospital had obtained at least 65 warrants over a 3-year period. Thus, a patient unable to pay a medical debt could end up in jail. In the world of consumer debt, even many creditor attorneys considered this step beyond the pale. Some of the country's largest commercial creditors, including Sears, Roebuck & Co. and the finance arm of Ford Motor Company, had a long-standing ban on the practice of seeking the arrest of "no-show debtors."[21]

Lagnado also wrote about other hospitals that sought body attachments. She spoke to county officials in Champaign–Urbana, Illinois, who were so outraged by executives at Carle, a nonprofit hospital that sought body attachments against patients, that they tried to revoke the hospital's tax-exempt status. A hospital spokesperson admitted that a waitress and single mother of two who was jailed by the hospital after she did not appear in court over a bill for care she received during a miscarriage would likely have qualified for financial assistance. Still, the hospital did not accept responsibility for the arrest. "There is only so much we can do for folks," claimed the spokesperson. In this struggle with county officials, the hospital prevailed and retained its tax exemption.[22] But not all hospitals escaped unscathed; the Illinois Department of Revenue stripped the Provena Covenant Medical

Center of its tax-exempt status for similarly aggressive tactics against uninsured patients.[23]

The stories by Bass, the subsequent research by Rollins, and Lagnado's articles in the *Wall Street Journal* spurred a broader re-examination of medical debt collection practices at YNHH and elsewhere. Clergy in New Haven headlined demonstrations, calling on executives to "repent." The SEIU put up a huge billboard so that drivers on Interstate 95 could see its message to YNHH: "SHAME."[24] Yale law students volunteering at a legal clinic worked with Rollins and New Haven residents to file lawsuits against the hospital, claiming that it "wrongfully took, obtained or withheld the property" of its patients when it garnished wages or obtained liens.[25] They sent formal "demand" letters, arguing that the hospital should forgive debts immediately, particularly as it had a donor-funded "free bed" fund with millions of dollars to help low-income patients access care. Elizabeth Warren, then a professor at Harvard Law School, approved: "The hospital thought it was safe squeezing poor families who didn't have the resources to fight back. Now it's going to tangle with a whole new animal—a student-run legal clinic."[26]

YNHH's spokeswoman complained that the hospital was being targeted by the union, and that "we are probably better than a lot of hospitals."[27] Still, YNHH canceled the remaining debt owed by Quinton White and promised to examine other cases of prolonged collections. White posed for the *Wall Street Journal* in the silk pajamas he had bought in celebration after receiving the news. He told Lagnado that although he was relieved, he worried about "other people in the same boat."[28]

Forgiving White's debt was not enough for the SEIU, either. The union wanted the hospital to forswear aggressive collection tactics, so it continued to heap scorn on YNHH in the press. Andrew Stern, the union's president, accused the hospital of "acting like a predatory lender and not a caring institution."[29] Finally, in November 2003, hospital executives promised to stop seeking to foreclose on homes and said they were placing strict limits on other practices such as putting liens on homes.[30] In the two decades that followed, YNHH tried to atone for its dismal reputation, donating money and vacant lots to Habitat for Humanity, along with hundreds of thousands of dollars to other efforts to end homelessness. Its executives said they were aiming to be a good community partner. In a self-nomination for the American Hospital Association's national award for community service, the hospital administrators wrote, "We must reach beyond the physical confines of our medical center and into the community."[31]

The efforts of the union and community activists also led to a change in state law. In 2003, Connecticut's General Assembly passed a bill that reduced the limit on interest charged on hospital debt from 10 percent to 5 percent and increased the amount of home equity exempt from seizure in the event of foreclosure from $75,000 to $125,000.[32] The episode had caught the attention of hospital executives around the country. A spokesperson for the American Hospital Association said that "every hospital has looked at what they're doing," and some "are asking some very tough questions."[33]

The politics of this moment were complex. The practice of suing poor patients proved abhorrent to a wide variety of actors. Center-right politicians objected to subjecting the sick to legal action in a moment of weakness for which they held no blame. The idea of the hospital as an institution outside normal market relations remained alive in their minds, even as hospital leadership and courts abandoned the notion. Suing patients also discomfited people of faith on the left and right, who saw in the practice a disrespect for the value of life as well as predation on the vulnerable. To more progressive voices, hospital lawsuits against patients were an object lesson in the evils of for-profit medicine and the vivid proof of the need for a single-payer health system. For them, this particular outrage opened a window onto a broader landscape of greed and ruin. Critical voices on the conservative side, on the other hand, viewed collection tactics like YNHH's as a more isolated problem in need of a focused remedy.

This dynamic was in evidence during a congressional hearing held by the Subcommittee on Oversight and Investigations of the U.S. House of Representatives Committee on Energy and Commerce in June 2004, a hearing spurred by Lagnado's reporting. It was chaired by Representative James Greenwood, a Republican who represented a suburban district outside Philadelphia. Greenwood remembered being upset when he read about YNHH's practice of suing patients: "I'd be riding on the train reading the newspaper and I'd pick up my phone and say 'hey, just reading an article about such-and-such, let's do an investigation,' and that's how this started."[34] He was upset when he learned in Lagnado's *Wall Street Journal* articles that many hospitals resorted to aggressive tactics against low-income patients.

Greenwood found these practices too draconian for a nonprofit hospital. He believed in personal responsibility, but he also believed unaffordable medical bills befell even the responsible:

> When people asked me why I was a Republican, my answer was always, "I believe that societies work best when people have maximum freedom and maximum accountability." . . . But I also believe, as a former social worker, that people should be as responsible as they *can be*. And some people are working their butts

off without health insurance, through no fault of their own . . . it was beyond their control. That was the cruel thing about it, you had someone who was barely scraping a living together, and all of a sudden somebody gives them a $20,000 bill and puts a lien on their house, you know, that's crippling.[35]

By the time his committee staff had completed 7 months of research, Greenwood had already announced that he would soon retire from Congress, and the hearing he proposed on hospital billing would be his last as chairman. He and his staff wanted to make this one count. Greenwood was proud of the committee's investigations of corporate wrongdoing:

We did some of the very first Enron hearings, we did the hearings that put Martha Stewart in jail, we did hearings on WorldCom, Global Crossing. I remember [then-House Majority Leader] Tom Delay came to me one time, saying, "Greenwood, why are you doing all these hearings . . . beating the shit out of Big Business?" I said, "Tom, if we are the party of business, of free enterprise, we have to make sure that free enterprise works. . . . And to the extent you've got these bad apples running roughshod over people, we don't look so good, right?"[36]

These investigations allowed Greenwood to change corporate practices without dealing with the logrolling and gridlock of the legislative process. So when the committee directed its attention to any organization, its leadership took immediate notice, and often changed course quickly to avoid further public scrutiny. Understanding this, Greenwood's committee staff wrote to the 10 largest hospital systems in the country to inquire about their billing and collections practices. They found out that Tenet Healthcare, the nation's second-largest investor-owned hospital company with 99 hospitals in 14 states, employed more than 5,000 people in billing and collections. Greenwood noted that by the nature of their work, these were 5,000 people "incentivized, whether it is through bonuses or salary or advancement, to put up the numbers."[37]

Greenwood, a former caseworker for a county youth services agency, was known as socially liberal and economically conservative, although this ideological gloss did not explain his fury at the idea that hospitals were suing poor patients. In his opening statement at a hearing focused on hospital actions against uninsured patients, Greenwood said,

Today in this country an average working man or woman treated at a hospital can be stuck with a bill that is double what managed care or government programs pay. . . . Then, to add insult to their injury, they are sometimes aggressively pursued for these inflated debts. The situation is unfair, and it is unjust.[38]

Greenwood wanted to focus on the high prices charged to self-pay patients and on the legal tactics employed by hospitals to collect debts. The hearing featured testimony from leading academics in the field, including University of North Carolina law professor Melissa Jacoby, who studied medical debt collection lawsuits, and Mark Rukavina, a health care advocate leading a group known as the Access Project. Greenwood stressed the need for pragmatic action. He did not want the hearing to focus on a longer-term quest for expanded government health insurance coverage, a more politically divisive topic. He said his aim was "helping real people right now" through "concrete action improving the condition of the uninsured and self-pay patients facing medical debts."[39]

Greenwood was gratified to hear the hospital executives at the hearing explain how they had, in response to the congressional investigation, changed their practices to make sure charity-care policies were clearer, to offer discounts on list prices to uninsured patients, and to move some collection to in-house staff to maintain more control over practices.[40] Trevor Fetter, chief executive officer of Tenet Healthcare, used his testimony to describe a new policy toward the uninsured that had already decreased litigation and liens against these patients by 90 percent.[41]

Greenwood was not an advocate for universal health coverage in the same way as Democrat Henry Waxman of California, another member of the committee. Yet on the issue of aggressive collection, their outlooks were aligned. Waxman was equally upset by hospitals "turning bills over to collection agencies who engage in practices of harassing individuals, garnishing their wages, going after their homes, freezing their bank accounts." He declared that "these practices have no place in this country when the debt is incurred because of a person's critical need for health care."[42] By any measure, Waxman was far more liberal than Greenwood. Nevertheless, they both saw in medical debt collection a cause for moral outrage and a need for change.

Some of the hospital systems whose executives were called to testify before Congress faced public criticism from powerful people outside Capitol Hill. One was a conservative activist named Kevin Brendan ("K. B.") Forbes, a colorful character whose track record made him seem an unlikely champion for the vulnerable. Although his mother was a Chilean immigrant, during the late 1980s Forbes declared at a city council hearing in San Marino, California, that the city was being "overrun by foreigners."[43] He had come to national prominence as the communications director of the

1996 presidential campaign of nativist Pat Buchanan. But in 2001, Forbes founded Consejo de Latinos Unidos (CDLU), a nonprofit organization advocating for lower hospital bills for uninsured Latinos. This was a strange and incongruous turnabout. All of a sudden, he was publicizing cases of low-income Latino Americans who had been pursued by hospitals for bills they could not afford. His campaign targeted some of the largest hospital chains in the United States. His group filed lawsuits against hospitals, aired television ads likening hospital pricing to Jim Crow–era racial discrimination, and demanded executives at Catholic hospitals "end the price-gouging and visit the confessional booth."[44] According to Tamar Lando, writing in the progressive magazine *Mother Jones*, this pressure campaign played a role in Tenet's decision to curtail litigation and lower prices for uninsured patients.[45]

The most intriguing part about Forbes' work may not have been his dizzying transformation from anti-immigrant right-wing mouthpiece to advocate for the downtrodden but, instead, his motive for doing so. His own explanation was that helping the uninsured was "in his genes"; he said he was inspired by mother, who as a social worker at Los Angeles County Hospital in the 1960s had helped families apply for Medicaid.[46] But to some observers, including Lando, the real answer lay in an old Latin axiom: *Cui bono?* (Who benefits?). Forbes' work was bankrolled by J. Patrick Rooney, who had donated $100,000 when the CDLU was just getting off the ground. Rooney was the founder of the Medical Savings Insurance Company (MSI). This relatively small company benefited financially from Forbes' advocacy. When Tenet agreed to lower prices for the uninsured, it translated into savings for MSI, which was small enough that its negotiated prices were not much lower than those charged to the uninsured. *BusinessWeek* reported that MSI made as much as $2 million from this change. Tenet also agreed to arrange speaking engagements for Forbes and to contribute to CDLU "to pay for KB Forbes' time and expenses." Forbes and his benefactor both stood to benefit from this deal as much as the patients on whose behalf he claimed to speak.[47]

There was another possible motive behind efforts of conservative activists to get hospitals to be more transparent about their prices. The insurance firms owned by Rooney, Forbes' generous benefactor, sold high-deductible "catastrophic" insurance policies. He also advocated for health savings accounts (HSAs), a proposal to allow individuals to save money tax-free to pay out-of-pocket medical bills. Rooney was one of many deep-pocketed, small-government activists who argued that this combination of high-deductible insurance policies and HSAs provided a "consumer-driven solution" to health care affordability.[48] They claimed that health care could be made to operate by free-market principles if hospital prices were made public. Americans would then be able to shop around for the best prices. After the popular outcry against health maintenance organizations (HMOs) during the 1990s, prominent conservative policymakers argued the best way to rein in costs was through the discerning, bargain-hunting, health care "consumer" whose high deductibles gave them "skin in the game."[49]

Rooney's effort had powerful allies. The Medicare Modernization Act, signed into law by President George W. Bush in 2003, allowed individuals and employers to set up tax-preferred HSAs only if they purchased health insurance with deductibles of at least $1,000 for individuals and $2,000 for families. Owners of HSAs could then invest the money, which would grow without taxes on capital gains or dividends.[50] After the passage of the Medicare Modernization Act, it was clear that corporate America would turn to Rooney's high-deductible plans, so his companies became even more valuable. In 2003, Rooney sold one of his firms, the Golden Rule Insurance Company, for $500 million.

Ruth Lande, who was an executive in billing at the Memorial Sloan Kettering Cancer Center in New York in 2003, remembers sitting in meetings with salespeople for high-deductible health plans, who spoke eagerly of their "consumer-directed health plans." Lande considers the turn toward high-deductible plans a turning point, a moment when billing departments started to face tremendous difficulty in collecting not just from the uninsured but also from the insured.[51]

Hospitals throughout the country complained that patients did not pay their high deductibles, so these plans were causing their bad debts to balloon.[52] But this did not stop the spread of these plans. Rooney's vision of "consumer-directed" health plans came to dominate the insurance landscape. Private health insurance had never been entirely protective against health-related financial distress, as lifetime limits, network restrictions, and cost-sharing left patients responsible for a large portion of their bills. In 2003, before the rise of high-deductible health plans, a national survey found that 25 percent of non-elderly adults with health insurance reported difficulty paying medical bills in the last year.[53]

But if health insurance never brought true financial security, the turn toward high-deductible plans left behind even the pretense of protection. In a study published in 2011, patients with chronic illnesses who were enrolled in high-deductible plans were more than twice as likely to report health care–related financial burdens, such as difficulty paying medical bills and having to set up payment plans, than similar patients in traditional plans.[54] High-deductible plans caused hospitals even more difficulty in collecting payments, and they pushed even more hospitals to outsource the work of collections or to sell debt outright. Hospitals were ill-equipped to collect so much of the bill from individual patients. These departments were, Lande explained, designed to go to "war" with insurance companies, which threw up bureaucratic obstacles to reimbursement. In this war, patients were an "afterthought," and few staff were tasked with collecting deductibles and co-payments from the insured and bills from the uninsured. Lande estimated that during the early 2000s, 85 percent of staff in hospital billing and collection departments were devoted to insurance reimbursement, whereas 15 percent focused on patient payments. Hospitals also had difficulty finding staff who wanted to collect from patients, a task that demands tact, persistence, and a willingness to make uncomfortable demands of sick patients struggling with other bills. When hiring and retaining such staff proved too difficult, many hospitals turned to outside companies. "That, to me, is the worst thing," lamented Lande, because collection agencies "don't have any connection to the community."[55]

The rise of high-deductible plans in the twenty-first century was spurred by the same imperative that had led employers to turn to HMOs at the close of the twentieth: the drive to save on insurance premiums, which rose, alongside soaring health insurance company stock prices, during the 2010s.[56] By 2022, 58 percent of private-sector workers were enrolled in a high-deductible health insurance plan. HSAs, for their part, became tax-protected savings vehicles for wealthy Americans and grew to hold $100 billion in assets.[57]

These plans brought a wave of new medical debt, which sparked more debate about how to address the problem, debate that would come to a head during the struggles over the Affordable Care Act.

PART III

The Recent Past and the Road Ahead

CHAPTER 5
An Incomplete Answer

We thus find ourselves at a crossroads: Health care can be considered a commodity to be sold, or it can be considered a basic social right. It cannot comfortably be considered both of these at the same time. This, I believe, is the great drama of medicine at the start of this century. And this is the choice before all people of faith and good will in these dangerous times.

—Paul Farmer, *Pathologies of Power*

The shaming of Yale New Haven Hospital (YNHH) may have chastened some nonprofit hospitals for a time, but it did not stop the rising tide of medical debt throughout the country. After all, the mid-2000s were halcyon days for debt buyers, as some of the largest conglomerates bought up huge tranches of debt with hopes of quick profits. Among academic experts in health economics and health policy, few were paying attention. Medical debt has not, historically, been a popular topic in the books and journals of these fields.[1] These literatures tend to dwell on strategies for cutting costs for public and private insurers: prospective payment in the 1980s, health maintenance organizations in the 1990s, high-deductible health plans in the 2000s, and accountable care organizations in the 2010s. All are variations on a theme: the need to save money for government and health insurance companies. This is, perhaps, unsurprising, given the sources of funding for the academics and think tank researchers writing the papers. But given the large and growing toll of medical debt, its relatively infrequent mentions are still striking.

A few legal and public health scholars swam against the tide and continued to study medical debt. Some, such as Elizabeth Warren, proved so dogged because they knew it personally. By the 2000s, Warren held an endowed professorship at Harvard Law School, but she had been born in Norman, Oklahoma, to a family that lived, in her words, "on the ragged edge of the middle class."[2] After her father had a heart attack, he incurred medical bills and was demoted at work. He lost the family Oldsmobile when he was unable to make loan payments, and Warren started waiting tables at her aunt's restaurant when she was only 13 years old.

For much of her career, Warren had studied the causes of bankruptcy in America, eschewing overly theoretical tracts and instead combing through court records and interviewing actual human beings. When she realized that many debtors were, like her own family, burdened by medical bills, she started writing papers with two doctors interested in the same subject: Steffie Woolhandler and David Himmelstein, a team of physician–researchers, were at that time on the faculty of Harvard Medical School. With their long hair and gentle smiles, they both looked the part of the kindly physician, or perhaps aging hippies (Woolhandler was, in fact, a dedicated activist against the Vietnam War before medical school). They brought the spirit of organizing to medicine, where they drew tens of thousands of physicians into Physicians for a National Health Program, an organization they founded in the 1980s to advocate for a single-payer health system in the United States.

Woolhandler and Himmelstein are also the premier researchers on medical debt and health care access. In the 1980s, their article on patient dumping had helped spur political attention and the passage of the Emergency Medical Treatment and Active Labor Act (EMTALA; see Chapter 2). In a series of studies over the next decades, Warren, Himmelstein, Woolhandler, and colleagues cataloged the rising tide of medical debt in bankruptcy courts. In 1981, only 8 percent of families filing for bankruptcy did so after a serious medical problem;[3] in 2001, medical bills contributed to 46 percent of bankruptcies;[4] by 2007, they estimated that 62 percent of bankruptcies could be attributed to either a large medical debt or lost income due to illness.[5] These medically related bankruptcies were now afflicting the middle class: Most of these filers had gone to college, two-thirds were homeowners, and three-fourths had health insurance.[6]

These papers set off a whirlwind of debate over the precise definition and frequency of "medical bankruptcy," sparking a long-running debate among researchers about whether these filers were pushed to file for bankruptcy because of medical debts or whether they simply had medical debts alongside other unpaid obligations.[7] This debate over causation versus correlation was, at times, distracting, drawing attention away from the larger problem of medical debt. Still, the influence of the medical bankruptcy studies on public policy was profound. In March 2009, speaking of the urgency of health care reform, President Barack Obama told attendees at a White House health care forum that "the cost of health care now causes a bankruptcy in America every 30 seconds."[8] When asked to support that statistic, the White House pointed to a 2005 op-ed by Warren in which she referred to her paper using 2001 bankruptcy figures. Her language differed from Obama's ("Every 30 seconds in the United States, someone files for bankruptcy in the aftermath of a serious health problem"),[9] but regardless, the team's research figured in presidential arguments for passing the Affordable Care Act. During an address before Congress in September 2009, Obama warned legislators that "if we do nothing . . . more families will go bankrupt."[10]

Several provisions in the Patient Protection and Affordable Care Act, signed into law in 2010, were designed to alleviate the burden of medical debt on American families. Before the Affordable Care Act, in most states non-disabled, non-pregnant adults without dependent children were not eligible for Medicaid. Beginning in 2014, people with incomes up to 138 percent of the federal poverty level would be made eligible for Medicaid by a blanket expansion of eligibility throughout the country. In addition, under the new law, young adults would be allowed to remain on their parents' insurance until age 26. Every other adult younger than 65 would be required to have private insurance, either through an employer-provided plan or a plan purchased on an exchange. Subsidies would be available to people earning between 100 and 400 percent of the federal poverty level. This piecemeal scheme aimed to approach universal coverage while promising the politically powerful private insurance lobby millions of new customers.

Overall, the Affordable Care Act did decrease the amount of medical debt in the country, but it did not do so evenly. Why the disparity? In *National Federation of Independent Business v. Sebelius,* a highly anticipated decision in 2012, the US Supreme Court ruled on the constitutionality of the Affordable Care Act. Most of the press coverage focused on the surprising decision written by conservative Chief Justice John Roberts ruling that the individual mandate to buy health insurance was, in fact, constitutional. But in another part of his decision that ended up being more important for low-income Americans, he also ruled that forcing states to expand Medicaid was unconstitutionally coercive. States had to be given the choice about whether to expand eligibility or not. And for many states led by Republican governors and legislatures, the decision was made not to expand, even though the federal government promised to cover more than 90 percent of the cost.

As a result, medical debt remained stubbornly high in the South, where in 2020 almost one-fourth of people had such bills in collections on their credit reports, compared to roughly one-tenth in the Northeast.[11] This regional difference was in large part attributable to the fact that most southern states had not expanded Medicaid eligibility using federal and state funding after the passage of the Affordable Care Act. In states that expanded Medicaid in 2014, new medical debt in collections fell by almost one-half between 2013 and 2020. In states that did not expand Medicaid, new medical debt in collections decreased by only 10 percent during this period.[12]

Hospitals and activists lobbied for expansion. Some governors and state legislators relented, and in other holdout states, elections brought new state leaders who favored Medicaid expansion. In other states, expansion passed by ballot measure. Although 25 states did not immediately expand Medicaid in 2014, by 2022 the number that had not yet implemented expansion had dropped to 12.[13] In these states, people living below the federal poverty level who remained ineligible for Medicaid fell into a perverse "coverage gap," where they made too much to qualify for public insurance but too little to qualify for federal subsidies to purchase private insurance.[14]

Deeply connected with these regional and income-based disparities are racial, ethnic, and life-cycle disparities. A 2018 survey by the US Census Bureau found that 27.9 percent of Black households had medical debt, compared with 21.7 percent of Hispanic households and 17.2 percent of White households. In addition, the census study found that households with children younger than age 5 were more likely to hold medical debt.[15] A nationwide study of credit reports found that medical debt was far higher in poorer neighborhoods. In the poorest 10 percent of zip codes by income, the average person had $677 in medical debt, whereas in the richest 10 percent of zip codes, this figure was only $126.[16]

These figures can seem distant, disembodied from lived reality. Yet for some people studying medical debt, the issue is intensely personal. Few people understand the costs of a cancer diagnosis better than Fumiko Chino, a radiation oncologist at Duke University who studies the "financial toxicity" of oncologic treatment. Even before she started researching the subject, she lived it. Her fiancé, Andrew Ladd, was only 27 years old when he was diagnosed with neuroendocrine carcinoma in 2005. A PhD student in robotics at Rice University, Ladd was insured. But his prescriptions quickly tore through the $5,000 drug limit, so the couple had to start paying out of pocket for his medication. When Ladd's medical costs exceeded the insurance policy's $500,000 lifetime limit, he was on the hook for all of his costs. The couple borrowed money and moved in with Chino's parents, but the bills continued. She remembers "the stress and overwhelming crushing defeat of these bills that would come in every week."[17]

The cancer center threatened to stop Andrew's treatment if he did not pay. The couple breathed a sigh of relief when Ladd was hired for a professorship at the University of Michigan. There he received better insurance coverage than he had as a graduate student at Rice.[18] But 3 months after starting this new job, Ladd died, leaving Chino with hundreds of thousands of dollars in debt. "I stopped answering phone calls from debt collectors," she said on NPR in a 2017 interview—at the time, she still owed debt from her late husband's illness.[19]

In the television series *Breaking Bad*, Walter White was not wrong to worry how his family would afford his chemotherapy, although cooking meth to pay his bills was an unusual solution. The Affordable Care Act did abolish annual and lifetime benefit limits in insurance coverage plans, but many cancer patients continue to fall into crippling debt. Nearly half of cancer patients report financial distress; patients who experience such distress are both less likely to adhere to treatment recommendations and more likely to die.[20]

In addition to expanding public insurance, the Affordable Care Act also aimed to decrease the financial burdens on patients through new regulations around hospital financial assistance. For decades, private nonprofit hospitals have justified their tax-exempt status with the claim that they provide care to all who need it, particularly the poor. But until 2010, they were not required to have any specific written policy regarding financial assistance. The Affordable Care Act was the first law to require each nonprofit hospital to write and publicize a Financial Assistance Policy (FAP).

The politics of this provision were, like much of the history of medical debt collection, complicated. The idea of mandating a financial assistance policy was a priority of Republican Senator Chuck Grassley, who had long criticized hospitals for exorbitant list prices and inadequate charity-care and had even held a hearing on these issues in 2006.[21] Health care reporter Dan Weissmann has chronicled how Grassley became interested in this issue after a series of lawsuits filed by Mississippi trial attorney Dickie Scruggs. Scruggs was, at the time, worth hundreds of millions of dollars, a fortune he had amassed after litigating a class action lawsuit against the asbestos industry on behalf of shipyard workers, and most famously as part of the legal team that had taken down Big Tobacco in the 1990s. He was also well-connected in political circles; his brother-in-law, Trent Lott, was majority leader of the US Senate. In 2004, in the aftermath of the YNHH stories and amid congressional hearings on hospital collection practices, Scruggs began filing class action lawsuits against nonprofit hospitals alleging that their miserly charity-care and high prices to uninsured patients violated their obligations as tax-exempt institutions.[22] Scruggs certainly had a point: An analysis published in 2000 demonstrated that 86 percent of non-profit hospitals enjoyed tax exemptions in excess of the value of charity-care they provided.[23]

Scruggs also shared a provocative theory about why hospitals spent so much money hiring lawyers to take low-income patients to court over such small sums. It was not, he said, so much an attempt to recoup costs from these specific poor patients as it was to keep poor patients out of their hospitals in the future. He claimed it was a ploy to deny care indirectly, to scare poor patients away from the hospital in an age in which, at least according to EMTALA, they were entitled to some modicum of emergency care: "You can't squeeze blood out of a turnip," he said in 2004, "but you can keep the turnip from coming back. This is a form of patient dumping. They don't want these patients coming back."[24]

Alongside the *Wall Street Journal* exposé of YNHH in 2003 and subsequent congressional hearings, this litigation led hospitals to briefly reconsider their use of aggressive collection tactics. Michael Barrist, chief executive officer (CEO) of NCO Financial, the debt buyer profiled in Chapter 3, told investors in an earnings call in 2004 that Scruggs' lawsuits against hospitals had, for the moment, changed how they could "use litigation as a form of collection."[25]

To Scruggs' chagrin, though, almost all the lawsuits failed because there still existed no legal right to charity-care. Far worse for Scruggs, in 2007 he was indicted for conspiracy to bribe a judge. He pled guilty and served 6 years in federal prison. But while he sat in his cell, the unsuccessful lawsuits he had filed years earlier bore some fruit. During the prolonged negotiations over the Affordable Care Act, Senator Grassley succeeded in inserting the provision requiring nonprofit hospitals to have a FAP. Although Senator Grassley voted against the Affordable Care Act, and voted in favor of its repeal multiple times, this provision would likely never have existed if not for his interest.[26]

According to the Affordable Care Act and subsequent regulations, the policy should clearly state the eligibility criteria for free or discounted care (most often in the form of a sliding scale) and the method for applying for financial assistance. The FAP must also be publicized to the community on a website, in paper documents available on request and distributed during the intake and discharge process, and in a notice included on all billing statements. In addition, the law mandates "conspicuous public displays" to inform patients about the FAP in public locations in the hospital facility.[27]

Ideally, these policies help low-income patients access charity-care. But the reality remains far from ideal. First, neither the Affordable Care Act nor other laws stipulate how much charity-care hospitals must provide.[28] Hospitals are free to decide at which income levels patients will qualify for free and discounted care. The amount of spending devoted to charity-care also varies widely by hospital. A 2021 study published in *Health Affairs* found that private nonprofit hospitals devoted 2.3 percent of spending to charity-care, a share that was less than that of publicly owned hospitals (4.1 percent) and even less than that of for-profit hospitals (3.8 percent). Among private nonprofit hospitals, more than one-third spent less than 1 percent on charity-care.[29]

But this fact only begins to paint a picture of the reigning miserliness. In 2004, a survey of low-income individuals in Baltimore, Maryland, found that 37 percent of those referred to collections by a health care provider were below the federal poverty line and more than 40 percent were homeless.[30] In 2018, 38 percent of households with children and with an annual income below $40,000 had at least one medical bill in collections on their credit reports (Figure 5.1).[31]

There are regulations that appear to require hospitals to do much more to ensure that they do not burden poor patients, but regulators have interpreted the rules to allow aggressive debt collection. In a corner of the regulatory code known as Section 501(r)(6), which is also a part of the Affordable Care Act, the IRS stipulates that tax-exempt nonprofit hospitals

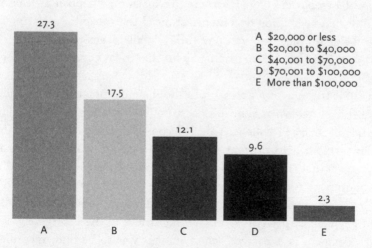

A $20,000 or less
B $20,001 to $40,000
C $40,001 to $70,000
D $70,001 to $100,000
E More than $100,000

Figure 5.1: Percentage of households with at least one medical collection on credit report in December 2018, by income.
Source: Octavian Carare et al., "Exploring the Connection Between Financial Assistance for Medical Care and Medical Collections," Consumer Financial Protection Bureau, August 24, 2022.

must "make reasonable efforts to determine whether an individual is eligible for assistance under the hospital organization's FAP before engaging in extraordinary collection actions against that individual."[32] So before a hospital's own collection department, a third-party agency, or a debt buyer reports a bill to a credit bureau, or a hospital denies further care or forecloses on a property, it is supposed to make these "reasonable efforts" to ensure they are not pursuing a patient who is eligible for assistance.

What, then, do "reasonable efforts" entail? As it turns out, not very much. After some deliberation, the Treasury Department decided that a hospital can be said to have made such an effort if it has notified the patient that they have an FAP, given the patient an opportunity to remedy an incomplete application, and processed any complete application to determine eligibility.[33] In other words, federal regulations allow a hospital to sue a patient to collect a bill even if the patient qualifies for financial assistance, as long as the patient has not successfully applied for charity-care. There is no positive obligation under federal law to screen for presumptive eligibility for patients who have not completed an application before sending the patient a bill or resorting to legal action.

But even this minimalist definition of a reasonable effort has proven too much for some hospitals. Administrators have gone to great lengths to prevent poor patients from ever applying for charity-care. In 2019, St. Joseph's Medical Center in Tacoma, Washington, settled a lawsuit filed by the state attorney general alleging that employees were told not to readily offer patients a charity-care application. If the patient asked for an application, the employees were instructed to insist on a deposit at least three separate times. Training documents showed that hospital registrars were advised not to ask, "Can you pay today?" but rather to ask more direct questions: "How would you like to pay for that today? Cash, check, or credit card?"[34]

In 2022, the *New York Times* wrote about similar practices at Providence, a nonprofit system with 51 hospitals throughout the Northwest. Seeking to increase revenues, Providence paid the consulting firm McKinsey $45 million in 2019 to help prevent low-income patients from learning about charity-care that the hospital was legally required to provide according to Washington state law. McKinsey developed training materials, which were used to instruct the hospital employees who were sent to repeatedly demand payment of patients who lay on gurneys in the emergency department. "Payment is expected," every patient was to be told, regardless of how poor. Training materials used quotations from Martin Luther King, Jr., to try to inspire vigorous collection: "If it falls to your lot to be a street sweeper, sweep streets like Michelangelo painted pictures." Providence used software from Experian to screen patients to determine if they were eligible for free or discounted care only after they had tried to collect payment for months.[35]

Perhaps the most knowledgeable person about the realities of charity-care is a former bartender and trampoline park manager named Jared Walker. After experiencing his own family's struggles with hospital bills, Walker founded Dollar For, a nonprofit that helps patients fill out hospital charity-care applications for free. His 2021 TikTok video, explaining how charity-care policies work and offering to fill out applications for anyone who asked, was viewed more than 10 million times.[36] When other people volunteered to help him, he had them collect the financial assistance policies of nearly every one of the 6,093 hospitals in the United States and used this database to build a screening tool to help people quickly find out if they were eligible for financial assistance at a given facility. By January 2023, Dollar For had helped low-income Americans save more than $22 million on their hospital bills.[37]

After assisting on applications for charity-care from hospitals across the country, Walker has found that they routinely require people to collect and print out dozens of pages of documents to prove income and assets. Then, patients have to submit the application either by snail mail or by a relic that few Americans have seen in decades: the fax machine. Patients might also be forced to undergo an interview with a financial counselor. Some hospitals, such as Centura-St. Anthony Hospital, a Catholic medical center near Denver, Colorado, even ask applicants if they have started a GoFundMe page.[38] "They're basically like 'Hey, if you're raising money on the side, we want to know about it, so we can tap into it,'" Walker explained. Even after going through all these steps, hospitals will often delay processing the application, so it is necessary to make frequent calls to check on its progress.

For many people going through medical crises, these are hurdles that prevent them from applying successfully: "Every little barrier that you put in, there is a drop-off," Walker explained.[39] He remembered one hospital in Colorado where the head of financial assistance admitted that the institution denied 90 percent of applicants for failure to show the correct proof of income. Other hospitals send out denial forms that announce, in bold letters, "You are denied financial assistance." The letter goes on to explain that the applicant needed to provide just one more documents, but some patients just read the headline denial, so instead of having their debt forgiven, they end up on payment plans.

There is, Walker explains, an easier way to determine financial assistance eligibility through software, which he illustrates through an example. For years, patients asked him to help apply for charity-care from the Oregon

Health and Sciences University (OHSU) Hospital, a large academic medical center in Portland: "Their application sucked. It was different from everybody else's, it was just, like, annoying. And we made a couple complaints." Eventually, the billing department started using software to determine a patient's "presumptive eligibility" for charity-care. Since the hospital moved to this system, where many eligible patients are opted in to charity-care by the hospital without having to go through an onerous application, Walker no longer receives requests from its exasperated patients.[40]

I spoke with two people at OHSU about their approach to screening patients. Kristi Cushman, Director of Patient Access Services, and Desember Terry, Manager of Patient Financial Services, agreed that before OHSU implemented its presumptive eligibility software, applying for financial assistance could be difficult for patients. "We had patients that would have been approved but weren't approved because they couldn't get us the documentation," Cushman explained.[41] More than half who applied for charity-care submitted an incomplete application, and went through a prolonged back-and-forth during which patients sometimes gave up.

Finally, Cushman said, the billing team came to a collective realization that "we've got to do something different because this isn't working." By 2017, they had grown tired enough of the "headaches . . . trying to keep track and follow up with all of these patients" that they decided to work with Experian, a credit reporting company, to implement a software program designed to determine whether a patient was likely to qualify for charity-care, and actively offer it to eligible patients.[42] The screening is not free; the hospital pays an annual subscription fee and an additional fee each time the software does a "soft pull" on a patient's credit report.[43] But the cost per patient is not high. "It's less than a cup of coffee . . . and I'm not talking a Starbucks," explained Cushman. The screening proved accurate; for 6 months the hospital continued to collect paper applications even as it used the software, and it found that the income levels obtained in both were remarkably similar. After they did away with the requirement for a separate application, this screening process saved patients from having to find and mail in paystubs and other paperwork.

Now, whenever a patient presents to OHSU's emergency department or an outpatient office and tells registration that they are uninsured, or that they will have difficulty affording their co-payment or deductible, a patient financial services representative receives a message. The representative then comes to the patient to offer to screen them for financial assistance and Medicaid eligibility. The representative runs the patient's name through the software, which, in a matter of seconds, pulls a credit report and other consumer data to estimate the patient's household income. If the patient's estimated income is low enough to qualify for Medicaid, the hospital staff will offer to help them complete an application. If the income is too high for Medicaid but less than three times the federal poverty level, the patient is informed that the bill will be covered entirely by the hospital.

With this change, so much of the bureaucratic rigmarole was gone. That is, Cushman explained, as it should be: "The last thing you want people to worry about when they are sick is the financial part of it. Let's worry about getting you well, and we'll try to help you as much as we can with the other part."[44]

Such software has been available for decades. As early as 2005, *Modern Healthcare* reported that hospital financial counselors could use a system sold by an information technology company called ADS Response Corporation, to determine patients' assets, income, and credit scores, and proactively determine who would likely qualify for charity-care or a state assistance program such as Medicaid. The software even partially filled out the application forms for this assistance. Reporter Vince Galloro noted that it could "avoid traumatizing low-income patients with medical bills that they can't afford to pay."[45] Despite its availability, 15 percent of non-profit hospitals do not report any use of presumptive eligibility software to the IRS, whereas almost 40 percent that do report using it also admit that they pursue patients for unpaid bills who would actually qualify for financial assistance. The most likely explanation for this, according to Keith Hearle, a consultant for nonprofit hospitals, is that these hospitals check for presumptive eligibility only after months of collection efforts or only on some patients.[46] So despite the fact that hospitals can readily access the information needed to screen patients, roughly half of nonprofit hospitals throughout the country bill patients who should, by the hospitals' own criteria, receive charity-care.

Even as charity-care policies have changed, lawsuits over medical debt have continued. To date, no researchers have been able to construct a national database of lawsuits against patients; court records in most states are too decentralized and too seldom digitized.[47] In a few states, though, comprehensive analysis is possible. In Wisconsin, hospital lawsuits against patients increased steadily between 2001 and 2018, rising by 37 percent; the share of the lawsuits resulting in wage garnishment rose as well.[48] In 2017, 36 percent of Virginia's hospitals garnished the wages of patients over unpaid bills.[49] In Connecticut, where activists drew attention to YNHH's collection tactics and changed state law, lawsuits against patients persisted a decade later. Between 2011 and 2016, physicians, hospitals, and collection agencies filed 81,136 lawsuits against patients in small claims court in Connecticut.[50] Between 2018 and mid-2020, one-fourth of the nation's 100 largest hospitals by revenue sued patients over unpaid bills.[51]

At the end of the 2010s, activists organized again to protest hospital lawsuits. Almost two decades after Paul Bass wrote about YNHH suing poor patients, another prestigious academic medical center became a target of protests for the same reason. And once again, labor unions were central to exposing the issue and pushing for change. In May 2019, the Coalition for a Humane Hopkins, a group that included the American Federation of Labor and Congress of Industrial Organizations (AFL-CIO), National Nurses United, and community organizations, published "Taking Neighbors to Court," a report that documented how, over the past decade, Johns Hopkins Hospital (JHH) in Baltimore had filed more than 2,400 lawsuits against patients.[52] Many of these patients would have qualified for charity-care under state law because Maryland required that medically necessary care be provided for free to patients living at 200 percent of the federal poverty line or below.[53]

The lawsuits were not financially important for JHH. The debts the hospital sought to recoup in court represented less than one-tenth of 1 percent of its operating revenue.[54] Maryland also had a unique all-payer system, which included a provision in which all hospitals contributed to the financing of uncompensated care across the state. Just as YNHH had a fund it could have drawn on to pay for charity-care, JHH had the benefit of ample funding to care for the poor without resorting to lawsuits.[55]

This was not a new phenomenon at JHH. In 2008, the *Baltimore Sun* published an investigative series documenting how JHH and Johns Hopkins Bayview Medical Center, another Hopkins teaching hospital, had filed 14,000 collection lawsuits over the previous 5 years. The president of the Maryland Hospital Association defended the practice at the time, arguing "nobody would pay their bills" without the threat of these lawsuits. Ronald Peterson, special adviser to the CEO of Johns Hopkins Medicine, told the *Sun* that if the hospital did not sue patients, "We could have bad behavior from people who are in that category of deadbeats."[56] In the wake of those articles, JHH did briefly slow the pace of its lawsuits, but only until the mid-2010s, when it abandoned restraint.[57]

Hopkins representatives claimed to monitor the practices of external collection agencies, but in practice, this oversight did not benefit low-income patients. Collection agencies contracted by JHH sent recommendations for lawsuits to the hospital, which were reviewed and authorized by an associate director of collections. The hospital's management did, in fact, know exactly who was being sued, and it was particularly careful with one kind of patient. If the collection agency recommended a lawsuit against a patient who JHH had deemed a "VIP account," the litigation had to be approved by a senior director. The hospital did not explain how it determined who was a VIP. Evidently, low-income Hopkins employees were not VIPs, as Johns Hopkins University and JHH were the employers whose employees' wages were most frequently garnished for JHH hospital bills.[58]

At approximately the same time that "Taking Neighbors to Court" was published, National Nurses United, the country's largest nurses' union, was trying to unionize nurses at JHH. Two months after the report was published, the coalition held a rally outside the hospital, demanding an end to the lawsuits. A hospital spokesperson complained that the union "sought to undermine the hospitals' standing in our community by publicizing misleading and unfair accusations about our hospital's medical debt collection practices." After all, she explained, patients were only sued after "more than a dozen contacts via mail or phone call along with multiple opportunities to file for medical or financial hardship."[59]

Change did not come immediately. Protests continued for years, but JHH would not relent. It took the arrival of the coronavirus pandemic in 2020 for the hospital to announce it would stop suing patients.[60] Not satisfied, activists turned to the state legislature to advocate for the passage of two bills. Advocates in the legislature recounted horror stories from Maryland residents. Lorig Charkoudian, a Democratic member of Maryland's House of Delegates with a PhD in economics and sponsor of the Medical Debt Protection Act, heard from one woman with cancer who was summoned to court to pay a medical bill. When she went to the wrong court by accident, a body attachment was issued. She was arrested and spent several hours in jail. "It is so absurd that that is the country that we live in," lamented Charkoudian.[61]

After months of intense lobbying by the activist coalition on one side, and hospitals and the debt collection industry on the other, the bills were passed. The first, passed in 2020, was sponsored by Delegate Robbyn Lewis, who had spent decades in international public health, including many years at Johns Hopkins, before becoming the first Black woman to represent her district in Baltimore Harbor. With this legislation, hospital financial assistance policies had to screen for "presumptive eligibility" for free medically necessary care—that is, free care without the need to send in an application—for patients who were ineligible for Medicaid or the state Children's Health Insurance Program but who lived in a household that received certain public benefits such as SNAP (food stamps), the Energy Assistance Program, WIC (the Special Supplemental Food Program for Women, Infants, and Children), or free and reduced-cost school meals. These provisions would help patients who were known to be eligible for legally mandated charity-care to receive it without having to complete additional paperwork.[62]

The next year, Charkoudian's bill, the Medical Debt Protection Act, became law. It forbade Maryland hospitals from garnishing wages, placing liens on homes, selling debt, and asking courts for body attachments and arrest warrants for medical debt. Debt repayment plans could not exceed 5 percent of a patients' annual income.[63] The bill did initially go even further, but a provision to ban lawsuits under $1,000 was stripped after lobbying from the state hospital association. Hospitals could continue to sue patients, although they would have to report the number of patients they sued every year to a publicly accessible state website.[64] Despite these limitations, these two bills had given Maryland patients the nation's strongest protections against medical debt collection.

While Johns Hopkins Hospital endured this scrutiny over its collection practices, another academic medical center was the subject of an investigative report for its aggressive pursuit of debtors. In 2019, a Kaiser Health News investigation found that between 2012 and 2018, the University of Virginia Health System (UVA) had filed 36,000 lawsuits against patients. In addition to wage garnishments, bank attachments, and property liens, UVA Hospital also made use of a state law that allowed it to seize patients' state tax refunds. Heather Waldron, a 38-year-old former nurse, was sued for $164,000 after being hospitalized for emergency intestinal surgery. Unbeknownst to her, her health insurance had lapsed before her illness. The hospital placed a lien on her home, which she planned to sell to pay as much of the bill as she could. She was living on food stamps and filing for bankruptcy.[65]

As at JHH, this was not an entirely new phenomenon. In 1984, the UVA Hospital sued the family of a dead boy named Richard Jason Oliver. Richard had contracted HIV through a blood transfusion he received at that hospital following a premature birth. He died of complications of AIDS at only 14 months of age. His parents, Lisa and Richard, had health insurance but nonetheless went into debt while caring for him and could not even afford a headstone for his grave. They did not know he had AIDS until after his death, when they learned that three other infants had also contracted the disease at the hospital. Dr. John Ashley, administrator of the UVA Hospital, said the hospital had not explained to Richard's parents that he had AIDS because it was "medical jargon" and "not appropriate for an infant." The hospital, however, did inform Lisa and Richard that they were being sued for $3,000 in unpaid bills. "As long as the care issued to a patient was appropriate and we can justify the charges, we're required to pursue the debt," said Dr. Ashley. Apparently, this was not a very strict requirement, as the hospital dropped the lawsuit after a *Washington Post* article on the Olivers' ordeal.[66]

More than 30 years later, media exposure did result in some changes. Days after the *Washington Post* published its first article on UVA Hospital's medical debt lawsuits, the health system promised to "reduce our reliance on the legal system." Specifically, it would not sue patients unless they owed at least $1,000 and their family income was above 400 percent of the federal poverty level. The changes were not retroactive, so would not automatically benefit Heather Waldron, although UVA officials claimed they were "committed to working with anyone who currently has an outstanding balance or debt that they are struggling to pay."[67]

But academic medical centers were not the only hospitals in on the act. In his book *The Price We Pay*, Marty Makary, a surgeon at Johns Hopkins, wrote about visiting New Mexico after learning about the practices of for-profit Carlsbad Medical Center. When Makary visited the local courthouse to look into lawsuits, the clerks were relieved to hear someone was doing something about the hospital. "They go after everyone," one clerk explained. "Old people, disabled people, people who can't pay, the insured, the uninsured. . . . They even garnished an old man's 401(k) retirement dividends." After reviewing court records, Makary estimated that one in five people in the town had had their wages garnished by the medical center.[68]

These lurid stories of hospitals' aggressive collections arouse the ire of people steeped in the idea of the hospital as a charitable institution. But to at least one expert on medical debt, Melissa Jacoby, the focus on hospitals as primary villains in this drama—common in congressional hearings and newspaper stories alike—obscures deeper pathologies in the political economy of health finance. Understanding the problem, she insisted, requires going beyond blaming the behavior of individual actors. Although she was among the first scholars to document the impact of aggressive medical debt collection practices, Jacoby has also long warned against a singular focus on "hospital misbehavior." She explained in an interview that she was "not an apologist for hospitals" and that "the hospitals deserved the shame that they've received."[69] But that shame could not be the end of the conversation.

A 2006 article that Jacoby co-authored with Elizabeth Warren argued for a re-examination of the broader system of health care financing and the burdens it places on patients and their families. As Jacoby and Warren explained, the high prices charged the uninsured, the stingy charity-care policies, and the aggressive debt collection tactics were but a small piece of the larger problem, and a focus on these items alone limited the reform agenda to actions such as Dickie Scruggs' failed class action lawsuits and minor, short-lived reforms in hospital billing practices.

Jacoby and Warren argued that focusing only on the tactics of hospitals—a "hospital misbehavior model"—left out a number of ways health care costs hurt families. The focus in the mid-2000s on the high prices charged to the uninsured ignored the fact that even insured patients were often in medical debt. The focus on hospital bills left out the burden of medical office visits, prescription drugs, and income lost to illness. Critics of their work said that they overstated the impact of medical bankruptcy, but these criticisms failed to take into account the way that medical bills coexist with other kinds of consumer debts. For instance, medical bills are often charged to credit cards, so court records of medical debt underestimate their import in outcomes such as bankruptcy. By 2008, an estimated $45 billion in bills for medical care were paid using credit cards and credit lines.[70] This was, they concluded, a complex problem requiring a much more robust policy response than shaming hospitals.

Even when narrowing the focus to hospital bills, "the problem is," Jacoby and Warren explained, "largely structural and not behavioral," so "legal and policy solutions to alleged hospital misbehavior are likely to bring very limited relief."[71] They objected to the self-proclaimed pragmatism of people such as Representative James Greenwood, who insisted while chairing the committee hearing chronicled in Chapter 4 that the focus should be limited to hospital practices rather than broader discussions of health care financing.[72] They noted that after the congressional hearings, class action lawsuits, protests, and newspaper articles of 2003–2004, hospitals had "furiously studied and vowed to change their billing and collections practices" through new state hospital association guidelines and voluntary restraints on otherwise legal activities.[73] But this frenzy of promises left much untouched. Complex Medicare law and regulations requiring efforts to collect outstanding debts caused hospital administrators trepidation when trying to craft more lenient policies.[74] State and federal laws continued to permit medical providers to pursue the same kinds of collection tactics (liens, garnishing wages, attaching bank accounts) as other creditors. It mattered not, they observed, "whether the debt was incurred for a trip to the Bahamas or to the emergency room of the local hospital."[75]

Legal precedent in debtor–creditor litigation gave hospitals wide latitude to collect bills, even in extraordinary circumstances when patients and their families were under life-threatening duress. For example, a 1993 decision by a Missouri Court of Appeals allowed Heartland Health Systems to collect an $8,500 bill from Andrew Chamberlin, an 18-year-old brought to its hospital unconscious following a motor vehicle accident, as well as from his mother, Iola Chamberlin. Iola had signed a consent form for his care without knowing she was obliging herself to pay for his bill. Iola had signed, she explained, "so they would give him medical treatment because he needed it because he was bleeding out of his ears, out of his mouth, the bone out of his elbow was sticking out through the skin." No matter, ruled the judges. Iola had obliged herself to pay for his care by signing a contract and was not, in fact, under duress when she signed it. Therefore, her ignorance of the content of the contract she signed and of the hospital's legal duty to stabilize her son's emergent medical conditions did not excuse her from her financial obligations. The court also ruled that Andrew was liable for the hospital charges, even though he had been brought in unconscious.[76]

Jacoby and Warren explained that hospitals engaging in debt collection were not only acting within the law but also responding to incentives and economic pressures over which they had little control:

> Hospitals have limited capacity to provide enduring answers. They cannot finance the health care of the uninsured even if they spend every dollar of the value of their tax exemptions. They already collect far less than the full amount from self-pay patients.[77]

Even if lawmakers sought to do nothing other than protect the uninsured from large hospital bills, they could not stop at shaming hospitals but would also have to change state laws that gave them (as well as third-party financiers of medical debt, such as credit card companies) rights to collect on these debts using aggressive measures.

The prevalence of the problem of aggressive debt collection and the extremes to which it is taken demonstrate the true nature of the American way of health financing, how patients are ultimately made to bear unbearable costs. They show how, in a landscape full of billboards and commercials professing care and compassion, even nonprofit health care providers can be ruthless in exacting repayment. This has led to some dour views on the purportedly charitable missions of these institutions. When University of Illinois law professor John Colombo testified before Congress in 2005 about the need for additional accountability to ensure hospitals justified their tax exemptions, he opined that "hospitals long ago quit being almshouses for the poor. Today, they are multimillion- or multibillion-dollar businesses."[78] It is difficult to argue that their actions do not support this opinion.

But if nonprofit hospitals failed to live by widely held ideals about their charitable missions, avowedly for-profit actors pursued debts without this historical baggage. A blitz of private equity buyouts of physician groups and hospitals in the mid-2010s brought a reinvigorated aggression to debt collection. Typically, a private equity firm uses debt to finance a leveraged buyout, then saddles the company it purchased with that debt. Over the next few years, it cuts costs and drives up revenues in anticipation of a quick resale.[79] When private equity firms buy hospitals or physician groups, their determination to rapidly raise revenues can lead to unforgiving attitudes toward patients in debt.

One of the best-documented cases occurred in 2017 when Blackstone, the world's largest private equity firm, purchased TeamHealth, an emergency physician staffing firm with more than 16,000 doctors, for $6.1 billion. After this buyout, one of TeamHealth's subsidiary firms, Southeastern Emergency Physicians, began suing patients at a vastly accelerated pace. Investigative journalists at ProPublica and MLK50 found that during the 2 years following the buyout, Southeastern filed more than 4,800 lawsuits in Shelby County, Tennessee, where Memphis is located. The number of lawsuits filed by Southeastern against patients in Shelby doubled in the year after Blackstone's buyout. In response to ProPublica's coverage, TeamHealth eventually announced that it would stop suing patients and touted a new FAP for the uninsured.[80] The journalist's pen had, once more, stayed the hand of an aggressive creditor.

Private equity was at it again 2 years later when Congress was on the verge of passing legislation to end surprise billing. In this practice, common in emergency departments, patients who received emergency care received large medical bills from doctors who were not part of their insurance networks. When they could not reach agreement with an insurer, private equity groups and other investor-owned practices issued bills for the amounts that insurance would not pay. Patients expecting insurance to cover the bulk of their costs found instead that they were liable for large portions of the costs out of pocket. The compromise negotiated in federal legislation forced doctors and insurers to accept a price, based on the median reimbursement for doctors in that area, to keep patients from being saddled with huge bills. Unappeased, TeamHealth (owned by Blackstone) and Envision HealthCare (owned by Kohlberg Kravis Roberts & Co.) funded a political action group called Doctor Patient Unity. This group ran an advertising campaign using television, social media, and direct mail to oppose the bill. Some of the material called the bill a "first step toward socialists' Medicare-for-all dream."[81] Other physician groups eschewed such heavy-handed messaging and supported a compromise, which eventually passed in 2020 as the No Surprises Act, in which rates were set by an independent arbitration process between physicians and insurers.

Throughout the country, debt keeps patients away from their doctors. A survey by the Access Project found that doctors sometimes refuse care to all family members until their past-due bills are paid. Fear of such humiliation leads many debtors to forgo needed care, even if their doctors have not yet turned them away. One-fourth of respondents with medical debt in a Kansas survey said they changed primary care doctors because of their debts.[82]

Some in the debt collection industry contend that hospitals and other health care providers bear responsibility for their billing and collection practices. George Buck, a 40-year veteran of medical debt collection who now represents ACA International before the Consumer Financial Protection Bureau, told me that hospitals could help by doing a better job screening patients for charity-care. He also said hospitals should work to avoid errors in billing codes that leave patients with incorrectly inflated bills, and they should also be more lenient in catastrophic situations.[83]

Buck said that although there are some bad actors in debt collection, the industry is now regulated by a slew of laws and regulations, including the Federal Debt Collections Practices Act of 1977 (FDCPA); the Telephone Consumer Protection Act of 1991 (TCPA); the Health Insurance Portability and Accountability Act of 1996 (HIPAA); and the Unfair, Deceptive, or Abusive Acts or Practices (UDAAP) provisions of the Dodd–Frank Wall Street Reform and Consumer Protection Act of 2010. These laws dictate how debt collectors use and share information and how they interact with debtors. Although they do little to limit the amount of debt a patient might be responsible for, or what legal tactics collectors can pursue, they at least aim to prevent overt verbal abuse of debtors over the phone. When collectors run afoul of these rules, they face fines from government regulators and lawsuits from aggrieved debtors.

Buck pointed to other trends that he said lead hospitals to rely more on collection agencies. Health insurance companies have turned to higher co-payments and higher deductibles, leaving the insured with a greater burden of out-of-pocket costs. As early as 2008, Trey Daly of the Legal Aid Society of Greater Cincinnati observed that a growing number of people seeking assistance after being sued by hospitals actually had health insurance.[84] In the decade that followed, the average deductible for a single worker tripled.[85] Employers seeking to cut premium costs and individuals purchasing insurance through the exchange with limited budgets both opted for high-deductible plans.[86] By 2017, the typical single American with insurance through an employer was responsible for $1,820 in annual deductibles.[87] These rising out-of-pocket costs for the insured left them increasingly vulnerable.

Even as millions of Americans gained insurance through the marketplace set up by the Department of Health and Human Services after the passage of the Affordable Care Act, high-deductible plans were allowed on the exchange, and the protection provided by the insurance coverage on offer was diminished by the fact that high-deductible plans were allowed. University of Pennsylvania health economist Mark Pauly argued that the mandate to buy health insurance included in the Affordable Care Act should, in theory, do away with objections to collection:

> So if you don't pay up, it means you chose not to have insurance and it's OK to go after you. . . . In real life, there will be sad stories, but as a concept we've taken away the claim that "I incurred this medical debt [because] I couldn't afford medical care."[88]

But in real life, health care remains unaffordable for many with insurance. Marketplace plans allow annual out-of-pocket spending as high as $8,200 for an individual. Jennifer Roulette, a lawyer at Legal Action of Wisconsin, observed, "We see medical debt collection against people who have purchased marketplace plans that don't seem to cover a whole lot."[89]

Buck argued that because of such structural changes, hospitals were increasingly desperate to collect unpaid bills. They turned to collection agencies that were themselves struggling with increasing competition and lower contingent rates. In the face of these pressures, collectors put more pressure on debtors by reporting them to credit bureaus and suing them in small claims courts. The onus, he says, is on health care providers who hire the agencies to "do a better job expressing what the boundaries are."[90]

Although it might be easy to attribute comments such as Buck's to self-interest, legal scholars also worry about reforms to billing and collection that leave hospitals, rather than patients, holding the bag for unpaid debts. In a 2007 article, Melissa Jacoby observed that most medical debts were not large enough to be considered catastrophic. She explained that because medical bills

> do not differ significantly in magnitude from debts arising from other necessities that result in debt on credit reports, such as utilities, shelter, food, and clothing, the justification for a legal distinction in collection practices becomes less obvious, particularly if the medical bills are arising from routine care.[91]

Restrictions on medical debt collection might lead "financially stressed" but "non-poor" households to "move medical providers even further down the priority list than they are today, leaving providers trying to adjust to greater shortfalls through, say, altering services or reducing charity care."[92] Thus, well-intentioned reforms might harm the finances of hospitals that seek to care for the poor.

Ultimately, Buck and Jacoby and all the critics of reformism have a point. Shifting the burden off patients, even temporarily, through restrictions on collection does not ultimately leave struggling hospitals with more money to care for them. Many institutions have long tried to provide care without sufficient state and federal funding to properly care for the uninsured and underinsured.[93] Many safety-net and rural hospitals exist on the brink of collapse, and some have closed their doors for good.[94] But the available data does not support the idea that hospitals with precarious hospital finances are those that try hardest to restrict access for the poor. An analysis of 2017 Medicare cost reports found that nonprofit hospitals with the highest net incomes (that is, the hospitals with the highest operating margins) provide far less charity-care, as a portion of net income, than other nonprofit hospitals.[95] Some of the most well-heeled medical centers with healthy operating margins make it difficult for patients to get charity-care, or even to be seen in their facilities. In the University of California Health System, specialists such as neurologists, orthopedic surgeons, and cardiologists do not, as a general rule, take patients enrolled in Medi-Cal, California's Medicaid program, despite the fact that revenues far exceed expenses at many University of California medical campuses.[96]

These decades-long shifts in public and private reimbursements and unaffordable out-of-pocket payments have made it more difficult for some hospitals to pay their expenses. Making hospitals foot more of the bill is not a viable long-term solution, particularly for hospitals struggling to stay afloat. But hospitals can lobby for funds more effectively than can uninsured patients, so cutting costs by limiting charity-care is an even more unjust answer to the problem.

There are people working to alleviate the burden on patient-debtors through piecemeal reform, while others propose to solve this problem once and for all. The former are an eclectic group with varied proposals that do not so much disrupt the status quo as render it slightly less burdensome for patients. The latter is a group of artists and organizers for whom the world as it is just will not do.

CHAPTER 6

Reformers, Abolitionists, and the Costs of Inaction

It is hard to let your heart break
every day, to feel yourself melt
into someone else's suffering.
It is easier to avoid sidewalk cracks,
to drink lemonade and ignore the
news, to dig a hole and crawl into it,
allowing only sunlight to reach your face.
It is easier to think not me, not me,
not me. Not me, not me, not me, until
you are not quite sure who you are at all.
                    —Hannah Rosenberg, "It is Hard to Let Your Heart Break"

When we were separate individuals, all we had was rage.
                    —Ray Bradbury, *Fahrenheit 451*

A movement was born, flowered, and then, it seemed to die. First in Zuccotti Park in New York City in September 2011, and then in public squares in cities throughout the country, millions had gathered, in a movement that became known as "Occupy." They were people angered by the fact that the government had bailed out bankers while leaving working people underwater on their mortgages, in debt to colleges and hospitals, and maxing out high-interest credit cards to afford necessities after being laid off. Organized along anarchist principles and using a process of modified consensus, the assemblies eschewed individual leaders, and sought instead to embody the kind of democracy they wished to bring about in the world. Although the movement was frequently criticized for lacking a discrete platform of demands, "We are the 99 percent" became a rallying cry that focused national attention on inequality and the capture of the political process by the wealthiest. In gatherings from Jackson, Mississippi, to Fairbanks, Alaska, Occupiers shared ideas in "people's assemblies" and books in "people's libraries," camped out at night, and planned direct action protests. Yet beginning in November, New York City mayor Michael Bloomberg and other municipal leaders declared the gatherings illegal, or unsanitary, and cleared the camps. But a small band of activists had been inspired, and they focused the insights of Occupy on the problem of debt, including medical debt.

In New York, a group of writers and artists helped bring new assemblies together to share ideas about how to move forward. In the wake of Occupy, this group started a collective known as Strike Debt. "Financial capitalism is mafia capitalism," they declared. "We are under no moral obligation to keep our promises to liars and thieves. In fact, we are morally obligated to find a way to stop this system rather than continuing to perpetuate it"[1] (Figure 6.1).

Thomas Gokey, an artist who specialized in sculpture, had read about the secondary market in medical debt, and he proposed to start Strike Debt's work there. Why not buy and cancel debt on this market? This would, Strike Debt members Andrew Ross and Astra Taylor hoped, expose "the seedy underbelly of the debt system and the inequities it perpetuates." It would teach everyday borrowers about the existence of this little-known market and demonstrate just how little the debt collectors hounding them had paid for their debts. Although it was never meant to be a long-term solution to a massive societal pathology, it was, Ross and Taylor explained, "a chance to offer others support and solidarity where the government has failed them."[2]

As it turned out, buying debt on the secondary market was no easy task. Gokey spent months on message boards searching for a debt broker who would sell him medical debt. But he was unknown in this world, where sales were built on relationships. The debt brokers did not trust him. "They were like, 'No way, you know, get away from me, dude,'" remembers Taylor, who is, in addition to organizing Strike Debt, a documentary filmmaker and writer. In November 2012, Gokey finally had a breakthrough. "He started calling and talking with one and got a bit under his skin. And this guy was like, fine, fine, give me $500 bucks," recounted Taylor.[3] For this price, they were able to abolish $14,000 worth of medical debt.[4]

With this initial purchase, Strike Debt had its proof of concept: It could buy debt in order to cancel it. It would do this not just to relieve specific

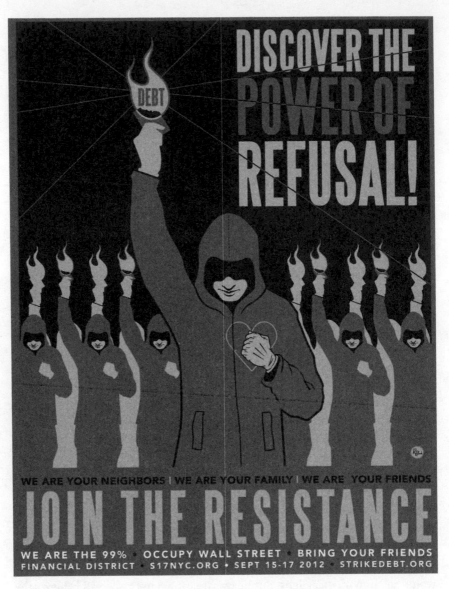

Figure 6.1: Strike Debt, 2012.
Source: Tidal: Occupy Theory, Occupy Strategy, September 2012.

debtors of an odious burden but also to spark debate about "the root causes of mass indebtedness" and the "coercive morality of debt repayment."[5] "A portfolio of medical debt is a portfolio of misery," wrote Taylor.[6] After their initial success, Strike Debt members aimed to buy much more of a commodity they thought should not exist at all.

The group estimated that with $50,000, they could buy and abolish $1 million in medical debt, while shedding light on the injustice of a system that drives the sick into bankruptcy. To their surprise, a viral social media post helped propel their telethon at a club in Manhattan (which featured standup comedians, lectures on inequality, and a mariachi band) far past its fundraising goal. By the end of the night, Strike Debt had raised almost $600,000.[7] Before they could use this money to abolish debt, they had to determine how to do so without running afoul of tax or legal regulations. The group spoke with lawyers, accountants, and debt industry insiders. "We had to master a field that was alien to us and that we were explicitly hostile to," remembers Taylor.[8] Yet if they were going to be able to buy enough debt to make some noise, they needed an insider's help.

In Jerry Ashton, they found a true veteran of debt collection. After completing Navy service and an undergraduate degree in journalism at San Jose State University, Ashton worked as a door-to-door salesman, pitching *Great Books of the Western World*. Eventually, he began to sell collection services to physicians for Transworld Systems, the debt collection company founded in Wilmington, Delaware, in 1970 that is now owned by Tom Gores (see Chapter 3). "I was a solution" for doctors, he explained: "'Dr. Jones, you know, you sent a bill [to your patient], and he didn't pay.' And [Jones] didn't grow up to be a bill collector, he grew up to be a doctor. And so he couldn't figure out what to do about it." The first of the services he would sell was "very benign," consisting of a series of letters sent out every 10 days. "They go out and say 'naughty, naughty, naughty, pay us.' And people would, you know, actually pay after those letters, because in most cases, people had forgotten about the bill."[9] But if the debtors did not pay, Ashton remembered, physicians' offices and hospitals sometimes turned to other, more aggressive collection agencies:

> They went into the hardcore. . . . These were guys with a fifth of scotch in one drawer and a .45 in the other drawer and they screamed and yelled at people and that's what people did at that time.

Ashton did not approve of these tactics. So in 1995, he founded a consulting firm called CFO Advisors. His firm aimed for a more "consumer-centric approach," trying to help in-house physician practices and hospital billing departments increase repayments before accounts went into collections.

Ashton was moving into retirement when he heard from Gokey, Taylor, and the other Strike Debt members, who told him of their idea. They wanted to start a "Rolling Jubilee," a concept derived from the Bible. In the books of Deuteronomy and Leviticus, there are moments of social renewal and debt cancelation among the Israelites every 7 years, and on a larger scale every 50 years.[10] Strike Debt's Jubilee would bring this concept into the present by abolishing consumer debt, including medical debt.

In settling on this idea, Strike Debt members drew inspiration from the work of one of their members, fellow Zuccotti Park activist David Graeber. Graeber was an anthropologist who had once been a professor at Yale University before falling afoul of the university administration for his participation in protests against the International Monetary Fund and the World Trade Organization. Graeber was a proponent of anarchist principles, which he described as "direct action, direct democracy, a rejection of existing political institutions and attempt to create alternate ones."[11] In interviews and books, he compared contemporary debates in the United States to crises in ancient Mesopotamia or the highlands of Madagascar. He was a playful and imaginative public speaker with a nervous giggle, and he was credited with coining "We are the 99 percent," the slogan that became Occupy Wall Street's mantra. Graeber's peripatetic mind, gentle demeanor, and humorous erudition endeared him to people yearning for alternatives.

Graeber wrote an auspiciously timed book, *Debt: The First 5,000 Years*, published in July 2011, 3 months before the start of Occupy. In it, he proposed mass debt cancelation:

> It seems to me that we are long overdue for some kind of Biblical-style Jubilee: one that would affect both international debt and consumer debt. It would be salutary not just because it would relieve so much genuine human suffering, but also because it would be our way of reminding ourselves that money is not ineffable, that paying one's debts is not the essence of morality, that all these things are human arrangements and that if democracy is to mean anything, it is the ability to all agree to arrange things in a different way.[12]

This call for a fundamental reimagination of social relations and widespread seething anger about the bailout of the banks ("They got bailed out, we got sold out!") were major motivations behind the Rolling Jubilee.

Ashton and another experienced collector, Craig Antico, helped the group buy medical debts on the secondary market. Ashton and Antico bought debt from buyers with whom they already had professional relationships. Then, the Rolling Jubilee members mailed out Christmas-themed letters to the debtors, announcing that their debts had been erased.

Most of the activists involved, including Taylor, believed this should be a short-lived demonstration, a popular education campaign to promote the notion that these debts could and should be abolished, that there should be a more structural solution to the problem of medical debt and predatory collection. They recoiled at the idea that it could become a long-term charitable endeavor, giving feel-good vibes to donors who forgave a small portion of existing debts while doing little to change the system in which those debts were accrued. "This is not something that needs to go on and on and on," explained Taylor,

> because we cannot buy and erase all of the medical debts . . . and ultimately there is a problem with subsidizing this industry. We don't want to be raising funds and then basically buying the portfolios of debt collectors that often can't collect them.

Taylor wanted to use the Rolling Jubilee as a way to "move people to the next level of engagement instead of doing this trick over and over again."[13] While continuing to write about medical debt, Taylor and her group turned their focus to organizing a union of debtors, the Debt Collective, that campaigned for debt cancelation; their efforts helped spur President Biden's decision to cancel hundreds of billions of dollars in federal student loan debt.[14]

For his part, Ashton did not want to end the work of the Rolling Jubilee. He did not aim to line the pockets of debt buyers, many of whom he considered "bottom feeders" and "scrap collectors." Worse than that, he explained, "there's human misery attached to [this debt] and they don't care." But he also thought their work was helping alleviate that misery for actual people, and he did not want to stop:

> Craig and I looked at each other, and we said, we can't let this happen. Because by that time, we were hooked. We read the letters. We knew the impact we had. . . . Our function was to right wrongs.[15]

In 2014, Ashton and Antico founded RIP Medical Debt, a charitable organization that used donations to forgive medical debt. The group received relatively little funding until 2016, when it was contacted by staff at John Oliver's HBO show *Last Week Tonight*. A staff member there had been given a copy of a book Ashton had written with Robert Goff, a former hospital administrator, titled *The Patient, the Doctor and the Bill Collector: A Medical Debt Survival Guide*.[16] Oliver's team asked Ashton to help purchase and forgive a tranche of medical debt for the show. On the evening of June 5, 2016, Oliver devoted an entire episode to the debt-buying industry. He described some of the most maddening practices of what he called a "grimy business," including threatening phone calls, lawsuits, and wage garnishments.[17]

Toward the end of the show, Oliver explained how his team had purchased almost $15 million of medical debt owed by 9,000 people in Texas. Then,

Oliver announced that instead of collecting the money, his team wanted to forgive it, "because it's the right thing to do, but much more importantly, we'd be staging the largest one-time giveaway in television show history."[18] He acknowledged that "much clearer rules and tougher oversight" were needed to protect consumers from predatory companies. "But, in the meantime, the least we can do with this debt I can't fucking believe we are allowed to own is to give it away." Oliver announced that they had directed the seller to send the debt to RIP Medical Debt, a nonprofit that could forgive the debt with no tax consequences to the debtor. "Tonight, at my signal . . . they will commence the debt forgiveness process."

Oliver promised that this move would "out-Oprah Oprah."[19] When, in 2004, Oprah had shocked 276 members of her audience by giving each a Pontiac G-6 sedan, the market value of her giveaway was estimated at approximately $8 million. The price of the $15 million in face value of debt that Oliver bought, on the other hand, was just $60,000, less than half a half-penny on the dollar.[20]

At the end of the show, Oliver pushed a big red button, music blared, and fake money fluttered from the rafters.[21] That night, so many people visited RIP Medical Debt's website that it crashed. From then on, donations poured in, from individual donors and church groups throughout the country. By 2020, RIP Medical Debt had purchased and forgiven $2.7 billion in medical debt, aiding more than 1.8 million individual debtors in the process. That year, the group received a huge boon when it received a donation from Mackenzie Scott, the novelist and ex-wife of Jeff Bezos, of $50 million.[22]

By 2022, Ashton and his allies were particularly enraged about veterans who are made to carry medical debt.[23] Although Veterans Administration (VA) hospitals were a valued source of affordable care, even they reported patients to credit bureaus if they did not pay their co-payments and other fees. This was particularly harmful to those who sought jobs that required a security clearance, because a credit check is a standard part of the hiring process for many of these jobs. In addition, non-VA medical providers referred bills to collections that should have been paid by the VA. These veterans were injured fighting for their country. That they could have their credit downgraded, thereby threatening their housing and employment, by their own government, for unpaid debts for medical care resulting from service injuries, seems a particularly grotesque form of national ingratitude. Eventually, the VA did begin taking additional steps to see if veterans were entitled to cost-free care because of disability before their debt was reported to credit bureaus.[24]

Meanwhile, press attention to aggressive debt collection continued to rise, with independent investigative journalists and public interest lawyers leading the way. In 2014, ProPublica and NPR found that Heartland Regional Medical Center in Missouri had been seizing the wages of thousands of patients, including many who qualified for the hospital's financial aid program.[25] Five years later, ProPublica partnered with MLK50 to report on Methodist Le Bonheur Healthcare, a Christian nonprofit hospital that sued its own low-paid, poorly insured employees over unpaid medical bills. The hospital sued so many employees that it became commonplace to see defendants coming into the courtroom after a shift still wearing their scrubs.[26]

The most aggressive tactic in debt collection, the body attachment, was the subject of an American Civil Liberties Union report in 2018. The report documented cases of medical debtors being jailed even when they had not been properly summoned and were unaware that they were being sued. Many were already desperate, and for at least one, jail proved one burden too many. In January 2016, a deputy sheriff appeared at the door of a 45-year-old Utah man named Rex Iverson with a warrant for his arrest. His offense was civil, not criminal, stemming from the fact that he had not paid a $2,000 bill for an ambulance ride to the hospital 2 years earlier. A collector had sued him in small claims court and, after Iverson did not appear, the court had decided against him by default. The collector attempted to garnish his wages, but Iverson was recently unemployed, having lost his job as a heavy machine operator. The collector then arranged to have Iverson summoned to the court to investigate whether he had any other assets to seize. When Iverson did not appear, the judge issued a bench warrant. Iverson, who had recently lost both parents in a car crash, was living alone in their home when the sheriff arrived to take him to the county jail. Later that day, when the police went to check the holding cell, they found Iverson dead.

After an investigation, the police reported that Iverson had committed suicide by strychnine poisoning.[27] This was a particularly excruciating means of suicide because strychnine, most commonly used in rat poison, causes involuntary muscle contractions so forceful that they destroy muscle, shut down the kidneys, heat up the body, and eventually make it impossible to breathe. Worst of all, perhaps, strychnine does all of this without affecting consciousness, so Iverson was awake for the whole terrible episode.

Such horror stories added to the groundswell of support for radical change. In 2019, efforts to go beyond small-scale debt forgiveness campaigns gained a powerful ally. As Vermont Senator Bernie Sanders stood near the top of the polls for the 2020 Democratic presidential nomination, he proposed a national single-payer health system as well as a cancelation of all existing past-due medical debt, which was estimated at $81 billion. Sanders said he planned to negotiate with the owners of the debt, although it was not clear what amount the federal government would pay for it. Craig Antico of RIP Medical Debt suggested that all of this outstanding debt could be purchased for $500 million.[28]

Sanders explained the debt cancelation plan was an attempt to right past wrongs, while single-payer "Medicare for All" would prevent any immiseration in the future. "We're addressing it on both ends," he said:

> We're addressing it now by trying to help the people who have past due medical bills. And we're addressing it by finally creating a health care system that guarantees coverage to people without any premiums, without any deductibles, without any out-of-pocket expenses.[29]

The *New York Times* noted that although Medicare for All had been endorsed by several Democratic presidential candidates, Sanders was the first to propose the abolition of medical debt.[30]

For its part, the debt collection industry has very different proposed solutions. These do not involve abolishing medical debt and tend to fall into the category of incremental, market-based reform. They propose to decrease the burden of debt on low-income patients without harming the profits of health care providers or debt collectors. One such proposal came from James Zadoorian, who has lived and breathed medical debt for decades. He worked as a lobbyist for the Healthcare Association of New York State, then as a business executive for a large nonprofit hospital in Chautauqua, before striking out on his own. As co-founder of TriCap Technology Group, he developed ARxChange, a platform that matched hospitals with debt purchasers. In trying to standardize the "complete Wild West" of medical debt pricing, ARxChange valued each bundle of debt by its collection potential.[31] This determination was based on a number of factors, including the age of the debt, the outstanding unpaid balance, prior collection history, the geographic distribution of the debtors, and the collection methods that medical providers would allow buyers to use. Potential buyers could then submit competitive bids.

ARxChange tried to replace the word-of-mouth networking through which debt sales were usually organized. Traditionally, hospital executives would sell debt to buyers to whom they had been introduced at a conference or by a friend over lunch. With ARxChange's platform, however, debt sellers could access a broader range of potential buyers in an online exchange. Medical debt could thus be bought and sold at more efficient prices, with agreed-upon collection conditions. Zadoorian argued that "by giving hospital executives more clarity and control over the debt sale process, they could also ensure that patients were treated fairly."[32]

The venture met with success. In 2012, 2 years after the company's founding, the ARxChange platform handled $9 billion in listings of medical debt.[33] By 2016, TriCap's other co-founder, Joseph LaManna, told a reporter that ARxChange was the largest analytics-based clearinghouse for medical receivables in the United States. Still, this business did not conquer the debt buying industry's imperative to network. LaManna admitted that many of the listings on the exchange came from personal connections the company made on social media sites such as LinkedIn.[34]

Eventually, Zadoorian began to proselytize another idea, one that he promised would simultaneously increase revenues for debt collectors and lessen the burden on patient-debtors. In an unexpected turn, given his last venture, he said he wanted to avoid debt sales entirely: "The need to sell receivables was a sign of failure, which meant that the volume of unpaid debt was high, leaving health care providers little option other than to sell their debt to recover what they could."[35] He noted that once bad debts reached the point of sale on his exchange, only 9 percent of amounts billed to uninsured patients had been collected, while 44 percent of out-of-pocket amounts billed to the insured had been recouped.[36] Patients were being handed bills, and many were not paying.

Instead of demanding every debtor pay in full, he said he could use big data (from 785,000 patient accounts and more than 200 facilities) interpreted through the lens of behavioral economics to determine just how much each individual debtor could be induced to pay. Specifically, in analyzing these data, he found that for most debtors, there was a threshold of debt repayment below which they would repay in full and above which they would throw up their hands and pay almost nothing. By optimizing for this maximum amount that each patient would pay, hospitals and physicians' offices could increase their collection.

Instead of using only income and family size to determine a sliding scale of financial assistance—that is, the standard way hospitals determine financial assistance—Zadoorian promised a system that was "supercharged" with additional data to arrive at a "revenue maximizing discount" for each patient. This would be a "fiscally responsive personalized financial experience," a form of "adaptive financial assistance" that would ensure the bill was reasonable enough in the context of a patient's specific financial circumstances such that they would pay it. Fewer bills would go to collections, and patient satisfaction would increase.[37] Zadoorian sought to distance himself from the "bottom feeders" who bought debt and ruthlessly tried to collect as much as possible. He went so far as to christen his system "compassionomics."[38]

But is it true that patients can afford whatever they can be convinced to pay? Many patients try mightily to settle their debts to health care providers. Fear that they will not be able to access care in the future, or of causing any strife with their doctors or favored hospitals, can be a strong motivation. There is ample evidence that patients take out credit card debt or even mortgage their homes to pay medical bills.[39] Demonstrating that patients will, at a given price point, pay off their debts does not prove that their financial health was not harmed in the process. Instead of asking patients to pay only what they can truly afford, it is possible that this initiative squeezes from patients as much as they possibly can pay until they give up on financial solvency entirely.

Other "outsourced revenue cycle management companies" promise hospitals that they can secure up-front payment, thereby eliminating the need to collect afterward. These firms contract with hospitals to offer interest-free medical loans to patients who agree to repayment plans. During the 1990s and 2000s, these companies usually decided terms of repayment only after insurance company reimbursements had been determined, thus clarifying how much the patient would owe out of pocket. The revenue cycle management firm would then pay the hospital the patient's portion of the bill, after keeping a percentage of that bill as a fee.[40]

During the 2010s, however, private equity firms made a wave of acquisitions, and the practices of these revenue cycle management firms changed. Hospital staff contacted patients before a planned procedure, or stopped by the patients' room in the emergency department following initial stabilization. During these encounters, hospital representatives gave an estimate of a patient's share of the bill and encouraged them to either pay immediately or accept an interest-free loan with a repayment plan. When the patient accepted the offer, they had to repay it in full, even though the estimates were sometimes based on the hospital's list prices, not the discounted rate negotiated by insurance. As a result, patients ended up paying more than they would otherwise owe.[41]

Laura Cameron's case, profiled in the *Los Angeles Times* in 2018, demonstrates how harmful these loans can be for patients. The 28-year-old librarian was 3 months pregnant when she tripped and fell in a parking lot. She went to the emergency department at Mercy Hospital in Rogers, Arkansas, for an evaluation. As she lay on a gurney receiving intravenous fluids, she was approached by a hospital representative who said she wanted to discuss how Cameron would pay her bill. The representative advised her that even though she had insurance, her bill would likely be $830.

The representative, Cameron remembered, was "forceful" and "made clear she preferred we pay then or we take this [loan] with the bank." Cameron believed she was not in a position to research her options—and understand the risks of these loans—while in the midst of a medical emergency. She declined to take a loan, and when the bill eventually came, she owed only $150.[42]

ClearBalance, the private-equity owned company that contracted with Mercy to offer these loans, calls its financing program "consumer-friendly" and part of its "mission of promoting healthcare affordability." Though such firms tout the fact that their loans are interest-free, this feature of their products can cloud their true cost to the patient. As Mark Rukavina of the advocacy group Community Catalyst explained, "If you pay 0% interest on a seriously inflated charge, it's not a good deal."[43]

When COVID-19 cases and deaths began mounting in the early months of 2020, lawsuits against patients fell precipitously. Among the 100 largest US hospitals by revenue, lawsuits fell by 89.9 percent between 2019 and 2020.[44] This happened, in large part, because courtrooms were closed. In addition, it seemed increasingly unconscionable for hospitals to sue patients when both their lives and livelihoods were, more than ever, out of their control. In New York, Attorney General Letitia James suspended collection of medical debt owed to state hospitals in March 2020, explaining that "in this time of crisis, my office will not add undue stress or saddle New Yorkers with an unnecessary financial burden."[45] She extended this suspension every month for more than a year, citing the "financial hardships of the COVID-19 pandemic."[46] Most major private hospitals in the state took James' lead and halted lawsuits against patients. But the state's largest health system, Northwell Health, was undeterred, filing more than 2,500 lawsuits against patients in 2020, even as it received $1.2 billion in emergency funding through the CARES Act. Only after the *New York Times* published a story about the lawsuits did Northwell announce it would stop suing patients during the pandemic and would rescind all legal claims filed in 2020.[47]

The level of forbearance varied widely throughout the country, and some institutions were unrelenting. Norton Healthcare, a nonprofit health system operating in Kentucky and Indiana, continued to file lawsuits against patients in the months after COVID-19 arrived in the region.[48] The University of Kentucky Medical Center stopped assigning unpaid debts to outside collection agencies, but those agencies were allowed to continue to pursue existing debts. "Unpaid accounts impact the cost of care for everyone," explained Kristi Willett, a spokesperson for the hospital. But the reality of lawsuits did not support any financial imperative for aggressive debt collection.[49] The Mayo Clinic, a not-for-profit in Minnesota, sued low-income patients in 2021 and 2022 and denied care to patients who had agreed to payment plans until their debt had been paid off, even though the total debts involved in a year of lawsuits would have garnered the hospital just 0.01 percent of the hospital's $15.7 billion annual revenue.[50]

Legislative attempts to expand protections for medical debtors during the pandemic proved unsuccessful. Senator Chris Van Hollen, a Democrat from Maryland, introduced the COVID-19 Medical Debt Collection Relief Act in 2021. This bill proposed to ban any hospitals that received pandemic-related federal aid from selling their debts or placing liens on homes, and it required them to allow patients on repayment plans to suspend payments. The protections were to last for the duration of the public health emergency. Like many worthy causes, the bill died a quiet death in committee.[51]

As public attention to the pandemic abated, the Consumer Financial Protection Bureau (CFPB) allowed collectors new forms of access to debtors. Starting in November 2021, collectors gained the right to contact debtors via email, text message, and social media, in addition to the older forms of telephone calls and postal mail. The social media messages did have to be private, although collectors could attempt to "friend" debtors on social media platforms. They could do all of this without the consent of the presumed debtor, although the debtor could opt out of such communication.[52]

At the same time, the CFPB announced a keen interest in the role of medical debt on patients' credit. A report released in February 2022 detailed how difficult it was for people to have errors on their credit reports corrected.[53] "Our credit reporting system is too often used as a tool to coerce and extort patients into paying medical bills they may not even owe," complained CFPB Director Rohit Chopra.[54]

The CFPB also detailed the widespread nature of medical debt, which appeared on the credit reports of 43 million Americans. Low-income families were harmed by having their bills sent to third-party collection, particularly because reporting negative actions on credit reports is extremely common in collection. More than half of collection agency actions are reported to credit bureaus.[55] Medical bills accounted for 58 percent of all bills in collections that appeared on credit reports. A decrease in credit score can increase the interest rates people have to pay on their mortgages and other loans. In some cases, it can cost the debtor a new job, as employers frequently look up credit reports during hiring.[56] The CFPB contended that medical bills did not reflect the general creditworthiness of a patient. Because they are so unexpected and uncontrollable, they are not predictive of an individual's general propensity to repay debts. For that reason, the agency argued, it would be more accurate to weight medical collection less heavily in credit scores.[57]

The same month as the CFPB released its report, the three major credit bureaus (Equifax, Experian, and TransUnion) announced significant changes to how they would handle medical bills. First, medical debt that was paid off would be removed from credit reports entirely. Medical debt would also have to be at least 1 year old before it could appear on credit reports (the previous minimum was 6 months). In addition, medical debts less than $500 would no longer be included on credit reports. These changes would at least limit the negative impact of debts, particularly small and short-lived ones, on patients' access to credit.[58]

In April 2022, Vice President Kamala Harris announced the administration's plan to help "reduce the burden" of medical debt. The Department of Health and Human Services would request data from 2,000 medical providers on bill collection practices. The Department would ask whether these providers filed lawsuits against patients or sold debt. These data would factor into the Department's decisions about which providers would receive federal grants. The administration also chastised hospitals and other health care providers that engaged in aggressive debt collection: "The federal government pays roughly $1.5 trillion a year into the healthcare system to provide patients with quality care and services," explained a press release put out by the administration. "Providers receiving that funding should make it easy for eligible patients to receive the financial assistance."[59] The administration also promised some medical debt cancelation for some lower-income veterans who owed money to the VA.

Although these policies could help improve knowledge about debt collection practices, and would provide relief to some veterans, they were not radical departures. In fact, Vice President Harris emphasized the administration's belief in the fundamental legitimacy of medical debt. "We should be clear: Most people with medical debt want to pay it off."[60] The Biden administration and executive agencies were willing to make small reforms to the system of medical debt collection, and industry insiders were proposing tailoring debt collection using big data, but neither called for the abolition of medical debt through a Jubilee and single-payer health care. Among people dissatisfied with the status quo, there remained two distinct camps.

After decades of ever more aggressive debt collection, is an end to medical debt possible?

Conclusion

It's safer to be cynical about attempts to create social change, and to list all the logical reasons such efforts will likely fail—to always bet on the status quo maintaining its grip. Activism requires a kind of willed hopefulness, a readiness to bash your head against a wall so that it may crumble or crack, even if you know all the arguments about why what you're doing is probably doomed and all the reasons the wall is unlikely to budge.

—Astra Taylor, *From the Ashes of Occupy*

In these days of hospitalization, I experienced once again how important is good health-care that is accessible to all, as there is in Italy and in other countries. Free healthcare, that assures good service, accessible to everyone. This precious benefit must not be lost. It needs to be kept! And for this everyone needs to be committed, because it helps everyone and requires everyone's contribution.

—Pope Francis, *Angelus*

When I first started thinking about this book, I thought it would be about medical debt in places that, to American ears, sound far-flung. My first book, and much of my early research, was about the history of medicine in Malawi. So my initial interest in medical debt came from coverage of the issue outside the United States. During the past decade, researchers and journalists have reported about poor patients being held against their will in hospitals in Burundi, Ghana, India, Liberia, Nigeria, the Philippines, Zimbabwe, and Uganda. Women who recently delivered babies, for instance, are held for weeks at a time until their families can scrounge up enough money to free them from the hospital. The hospital as detention facility was, it seemed to me, a problem worth understanding, if only to abolish it sooner.[1]

But then I came across cases of what sounded a lot like hospital detention much closer to home. Stories such as Ms. Wilson's, recounted in the Introduction, of people working as indentured servants in hospitals to pay off bills, often for dead spouses, opened my eyes to the fact that the United States has long been an epicenter of extraordinary tactics to collect medical debts. As I recount in the Afterword, I eventually found out that my own hospital was suing poor patients, garnishing wages, and cajoling people living on meager incomes to accept onerous payment plans. My once-global history of debt collection could start right at my hospital's doorstep.

As I discovered just how widespread aggressive collection tactics are, and how long debt collectors have been a plague on patients, I could not help but wonder: Where are the doctors? Whereas National Nurses Union was central to the fight to stop Johns Hopkins Hospital from suing patients, physicians' organizations were not nearly so involved. There are, of course, doctors crusading against this problem, in particular the tens of thousands of members of Physicians for a National Health Program who are calling for single-payer health care. And when informed about their own hospitals' practices, doctors usually express solidarity with patients. But with the exception of the periodic waves of short-lived interest in the issue, medical journals are not filled with stories and data about medical debt.

Part of the issue is that most of us have very little to do with collection. We do not know the charges for our services, and we do not see patients' bills. Physicians are busy enough with patient care and mounting bureaucratic demands. Many of us have no idea what kinds of collection practices our hospitals resort to, or the ins and outs of our financial assistance policies. We have, at most, a few hours of lectures on health financing in medical school; in my medical training, no instructor ever discussed collection practices. Hospitals are not eager to share this information with physicians, particularly when the methods are harsh and assistance is paltry. When Marty Makary, the Johns Hopkins surgeon and writer, asked doctors at Carlsbad Medical Center about their hospital's practice of regularly suing and garnishing the wages of their patients, "they had no idea their patients were being sued. When I showed the doctors what I had learned about the predatory billing practices, they said they detested what was happening."[2] When they heard what their hospital was doing, many of the doctors shared a sense of moral outrage.

Should we use this widespread ignorance as an excuse? No—particularly when our patients are being harmed by actions that result from our care. As former New York City Health Commissioner Dave Chokshi and medical student Adam Beckman argued, hospitals should treat lawsuits against patients and spending less on community benefits than they receive in tax breaks as "never events." This is a designation previously assigned to such errors as leaving a sponge in a patient's abdomen after surgery or operating on the wrong limb, preventable but immensely harmful events that patient safety advocates (including physicians) have studied and for which procedures have been devised to try to eradicate them from medical practice.[3]

There is, however, a reason aside from ignorance that doctors have been relatively absent from this debate. The physician as an independent professional is becoming a distant memory, seen in old television shows but rarely in real life. Although there are still private practices, many have been bought out by hospital systems and, more recently, private equity groups. Between 1983 and 2014, the percentage of physicians in solo practice in the United States declined from 41 percent to 17 percent.[4] For hospital-based doctors (like me), direct employment by the hospital or a physician group contracted by the hospital is typical. By 2022, 74 percent of physicians were employed by hospitals, health systems, and other corporate entities, including private equity firms and health insurers.[5]

We are no longer the masters of our own destiny. Particularly early in our careers, we are dependent on our employers if we want to pay back six-figure medical school loans. In exchange for freedom from this debt and the promise of later comforts, we become part of the machinery of the credit industry. In place of healing and liberation, we become unwitting agents of social control. If we are willing to stomach working for a private equity–owned or for-profit facility, our pay is likely to be higher. In exchange, we agree, at least tacitly, to keep complaints out of the public square. Increasingly, this agreement is no longer even tacit, as physicians found during the early days of the COVID-19 pandemic, when some who spoke out about unsafe working conditions were summarily fired.[6]

In 1948, the former coal miner and labor organizer Aneurin Bevan was asked how, during his tenure as the Minister of Health in the United Kingdom, he had convinced reluctant doctors to sign up for the government-run National Health Service (NHS): "I had to stuff their mouths with gold," he said.[7] Elaborating, he explained how he allowed specialists to keep seeing private-pay patients as long as they also took NHS patients. American physicians today have also had our mouths stuffed with gold, though not by the government and for less noble ends.

But now is the time to choose: Do we want to be in league with debt collectors or with patients? Debt collectors are not evil villains, but their natural incentives are antagonistic to those of people in debt. Every dollar they extract from the patient on the other end of the phone, or sitting across from them in a courtroom, is a dollar that patient will not have to pay their rent, feed their children, or buy their medicine. We have to ask, in short, whether we want to be allied with predator or prey.

After all, what is medicine about? That was the question posed by physician and social theorist Richard Gunderman in his 1998 essay, "Medicine and the Pursuit of Wealth": "Is it about maximizing the incomes of physicians or health care organizations?" he asked.

> Do patients and their suffering exist in some fundamental sense for the benefit of the physician, the hospital, or the stockholder? Or do physicians and the entire medical enterprise of which they are a part exist for the benefit of patients and the relief of human suffering?[8]

Gunderman argued that medicine was about the relief of suffering and not about anyone else's profit. This fundamental tension between widely held ideals of the aims of medical care and the market fundamentalism that dominates American life leaves those of us who work in health care with a gnawing sense that we are being drawn away from our raison d'être. It is the source of much disillusionment within medicine.

It is tempting to blame this all on our bosses. When we see the stories of hospitals suing patients, physicians and other health care providers I have spoken to often fault the highly paid executives who, we imagine, sit in meetings, gaze at spreadsheets, and rarely treat patients. But although there is undoubtedly truth to the charge that these C-suite executives have, in this history, frequently seemed to act with callous disregard for poor patients, we would do well to remember Jacoby and Warren's warning against relying on a "hospital misbehavior" model.[9] Their argument that this framing of the problem was insufficient proved prescient: Following wide publicity about hospital debt collection during the mid-2000s, lawsuits against patients continued, and even accelerated. This was, in large part, due to the refusal of some state governments to expand Medicaid after the passage of the Affordable Care Act and the rise of high-deductible health plans. Aggressive hospital collection tactics were never solely, or even primarily, a behavioral problem to be blamed on greedy and uncaring executives but, rather, a symptom of a structural malady. Liberals and conservatives alike make a mistake when they privilege individual agency and personal blame. Like everyone else, hospital executives and debt collectors respond to systemic material incentives. If these specific individuals do not pursue patients with aggressive tactics, surely some other individuals will fill their roles. The problem does not reside, then, within immoral individuals. Protecting patients requires changing the system that furnishes incentives to put patients in debt and then hounds them for repayment.

Jacoby and Warren were correct that the proposed solutions of the mid-2000s were inadequate, and the villainous portrayals of nonprofit hospitals might have masked a deeper pathology. Broader discussions of health care financing have to happen if we are to protect patients from financial and legal ruin. Yet the impetus to solve the problem must also come from real people's stories, from the pragmatic and humane desire to prevent suffering in the here and now. In this, both reformists such as James Greenwood and Jerry Ashton and abolitionists such as Astra Taylor and Bernie Sanders can find some agreement. Medical debt and aggressive debt collection are, to be sure, pieces of a broader tapestry of injustice. But they are particularly ugly. They rouse the conscience of most everyone.

So far, legislative action to address debt collection has focused mainly on preventing "abusive practices," a statutory definition that includes incessant phone calls late at night and failure to confirm a disputed debt. Meanwhile, the most outrageous burdens inflicted by our system of medical debt—lawsuits, garnished wages, foreclosed homes, even imprisonment—remain legal. After organized protest, some states, such as Maryland, have passed laws that regulate these practices, but for the most part the practices remain intact.[10] A few hospital systems, including nonprofit Ochsner Health in Louisiana and the University of Vermont Medical Center, have voluntarily banned lawsuits against patients.[11] But at many institutions throughout the country, the greatest harms to health remain, including the non-emergent care denied patients who cannot pay their doctors and care forgone for fear of debt.

Although the expansion of Medicaid in many—although still not all—states has helped lessen the burden of medical debt for some, countervailing trends such as the rise in out-of-pocket costs for the insured increase them for others. The debate about what to do about medical debt usually splits people into two camps. One camp favors the continuation of some out-of-pocket payments for medical care; the other opposes these payments outright. The former group may lament predatory tactics against vulnerable patients, but in the end, they contend that people should pay for the care they receive. The latter group points to every other industrialized country, where point-of-care payments are either nonexistent or minimal. In all of these countries, significant medical debts are almost unheard of.[12]

Now it is time for me to lay my cards on the table: I am against out-of-pocket medical costs. Arguments that co-payments and other out-of-pocket payments limit moral hazard, and cause people to decrease only unnecessary care, have not been borne out by the evidence. In fact, an analysis of cost-sharing in Medicare's prescription drug benefit program showed that an increase in out-of-pocket spending of $10.40 per drug caused a whopping 32.7 percent increase in mortality, as patients cut back on life-saving medicines such as statins and antihypertensives.[13] When patients are made to pay at the point of care, lives are lost.

Health care does not operate according to the expectations of a free market filled with economically rational actors. This fact has been known for decades, at least since Nobel Prize–winning economist Kenneth Arrow published "Uncertainty and the Welfare Economics of Medical Care" in 1963. This article, widely considered the founding text of health economics, showed how the usual assumptions of competitive free markets do not apply to medical care: Patients and doctors have unequal information, occupational licensing limits entry for "producers," and the social obligations of physicians push them to eschew profit maximization.[14] Thus, the impossibility of making health care conform to the assumptions of microeconomic theory was established in the mid-twentieth century, and the attempts that followed to make it fit into free-market ideals were misguided at best. On the other hand, the idea that we as a society have an obligation to provide care without ruining people financially is shared among people with otherwise divergent ideologies. This is at least a basis for moving forward.

Some proposed solutions would make incremental steps toward helping some low-income patients, but they are costly and byzantine. As shown in Chapter 6, no-interest payment plans offered at the point of care overestimate how much patients have to pay and lock them in to those high amounts. The adaptive financial assistance proposed by James Zadoorian, which tailors payment to predicted propensity to pay, promises to increase hospital revenues while lowering patient bills, yet might induce patients with enough guilt but little money to charge debts to credit cards. Propensity to pay and ability to pay without harm to financial health are two different things.

The process of applying for charity-care can be made much easier for patients and hospitals through the use of software to determine presumptive eligibility, although this usually requires hospitals to pay credit bureaus and other companies for access to consumer data. Advocates have long asked hospitals to emulate institutions such as Cooley Dickinson Hospital in Northampton, Massachusetts, where case managers help uninsured admitted patients fill out applications for Medicaid or hospital financial assistance.[15]

In the end, though, solving the problem of medical debt is not a mystery. To immediately relieve patients of the burdens of existing arrears, their debt can be forgiven, as the Rolling Jubilee showed a decade ago. The federal government could offer some reasonable settlement to the holders of that debt without making much of a dent in the budget.[16] In some places, such large-scale publicly funded debt forgiveness is already happening: Using funds provided to local governments in the American Rescue Plan Act of 2021, Cook County, Illinois (home of Chicago), and the city of Toledo, Ohio, are working with RIP Medical Debt to buy and forgive the medical debts of local residents.[17] But that is not enough; a lasting transformation of our system of health financing is needed to prevent patients from falling into medical debt all over again. As Astra Taylor explained, "We know that even if we could make all this debt dissolve overnight, the underlying dynamic that puts people into such a state would remain unchanged, and that they would just start moving steadily back into the red"; because of this, she continued, "What we ultimately need is a Jubilee—a cancelation of debts—coupled with a profound economic transformation that addresses the underlying causes and conditions."[18]

In 1942, the British economist William Beveridge called for comprehensive national health insurance, free at the point of care; his call still rings true.[19] Even those nations that do not have a single-payer system place tight limits on out-of-pocket spending expected from patients. The alternative is what physician-anthropologist Paul Farmer called the "OOPS" (out-of-pocket spending) approach to health financing, which is, as he detailed through numerous ethnographic accounts, a source of "despair" and "destitution" for patients.[20] Every year, 150 million people worldwide are pushed into poverty by out-of-pocket health care costs.[21] As a result, many avoid formal health care. For this reason, Farmer warned of "the mortal drama of any kind of out-of-pocket expenditure for catastrophic illness."[22]

Many countries outside the United States point the way. A variety of national health care systems have been devised and implemented that do not cause patients to fall into debilitating debt. Universal health insurance programs exist in every member country of the Organisation for Economic Co-operation and Development (OECD), a group of developed nations—every member, that is, save one, the United States.[23] Many, though not all, have instituted single-payer health care, in which all health care costs are paid by a single public entity, thereby eliminating the expensive and superfluous middleman of private health insurance companies.

Although many other nations have largely eliminated the problem of medical debt, that scourge is, even to citizens of those countries, a living memory. Margaret Atwood recounted that in the days after her brother was born in Montreal in 1957, her father struggled to free her mother from the hospital. He had not yet received his monthly paycheck, and the hospital demanded payment in full prior to discharge. This was the same kind of hospital detention now seen in some parts of Africa and Asia. In Atwood's words, Canadian hospitals had, at that time, "a lot in common with debtors' prisons."[24] Even after receiving his wages, her father could barely afford the bill to liberate his wife and infant son.

No longer. Today, Canadian citizens pay no money at all for hospitalizations.[25] In Germany, a patient is charged nothing to visit a physician.[26] A survey of OECD countries found that the United States had by far the greatest burden of health care bills on individuals, with 7.4 percent of its residents facing catastrophic health care bills each year. In a distant second place, Australia had a rate of 3.2 percent. Most other countries were far lower: Japan was 2.6 percent, France 1.9 percent, Germany 1.4 percent, and the Netherlands 1.1 percent.[27] As one UK resident explained of the NHS, "There are no bills, no paperwork, no deductibles, no insurance companies to deal with, no 'patient statements,' no risk of going bankrupt if you get the 'wrong' disease."[28] A 2022 survey found that whereas only 35 percent of Americans had a positive view of their own health system, 78 percent of Britons approved of the NHS.[29] This disparity in satisfaction is particularly striking because Britons have bemoaned inadequate health funding by recent UK governments.

In the United States, the struggle to forge a system that does not impoverish patients has been going on for more than a century, and continues still. "Medicare for All" is a new slogan for a national single-payer health care system, but it is not a new idea. Publicly financed national health insurance is an idea with a long history in the United States. It has, at many points, come tantalizingly close to realization. Although it remains elusive, it has long been popular. Even in 1982, at the zenith of Reagan-era go-go individualism, a national survey found a plurality of Americans in favor of a "government health insurance plan that would pay for most forms of health insurance and would be financed by tax money." A majority of respondents stated they would be more likely to vote for a candidate who "supported an all-inclusive government sponsored national health insurance program."[30] In recent years, Medicare for All has been endorsed by some of the largest associations of medical and public health professionals in the country, including the American Public Health Association, the American College of Physicians, and National Nurses United.[31] Single-payer health care is, as President Barack Obama admitted in 2008, the most rational way to pay for health care.[32]

Still, this kind of transformation is often dismissed as a pipe dream. Proponents of more incremental reform have argued it is counterproductive to focus on this goal given the powerful special interests—namely health insurance companies, pharmaceutical companies, and risk-averse voters who have relatively good insurance coverage—that oppose it.[33] It is absolutely true that single-payer health care legislation would not be easy to pass. The history of similar legislation, in the United States and abroad, demonstrates as much. In the United Kingdom, the Labour Party inaugurated the NHS in 1948 even as the president of the British Hospital Association accused the government of "mass murder."[34] In the Canadian province of Saskatchewan in 1962, doctors went on strike after Tommy Douglas' socialist government introduced a single-payer healthcare system. The system endured, and within a decade, the entire country had universal publicly administered health insurance.[35]

Change has never been easy in the United States, either. Medicare, a form of national health insurance for America's elderly, faced bitter opposition. In a recording commissioned by the American Medical Association in the early 1960s, then-actor and conservative activist Ronald Reagan declared that a bill introduced by Rhode Island Congressman Aime Forand, which was a precursor to Medicare, would bring an end to American liberty. Reagan warned that if Americans did not contact their members of Congress en masse to stop the passage of the bill, "one of these days you and I are going to spend our sunset years telling our children, and our children's children, what it once was like in America when men were free." In 2021, 94 percent of Americans with Medicare coverage reported being satisfied with the quality of their medical care, and a far smaller portion of America's elderly faced financial distress as a result of medical bills than did non-elderly adults.[36]

Only half of the states chose to expand Medicaid in 2014, even though the federal government was paying the vast majority of the costs. Due in large part to grassroots campaigns and ballot initiatives, half of the holdout states expanded Medicaid eligibility by 2022. This expansion in public insurance led to steep declines in medical debt. Programs such as Medicare and Medicaid that take the financial burden off patients faced significant hurdles to passage, but today they are widely popular.

Prognosticators and pundits often deem political transformations (for better and worse) impossible until the moment they become reality. The study of history does not vindicate cynicism. Our impoverished political imaginaries serve only to further entrench the status quo, when so much more is possible. No one has fated hospitals in America to be palaces of plunder; they can be houses of healing.

AFTERWORD

My Day in Court

The suffering and often disabled patient need not approach the physician with the motto of the marketplace foremost in mind—Caveat Emptor, "buyer beware." They believe that, in contrast to the used car salesman, they can trust their doctor to do what is best for them.

—Richard Gunderman, "Medicine and the Pursuit of Wealth"

The Governor Philip W. Noel Judicial Complex appears out of place. Its five-story edifice, with walls of brick and glass and an elegantly recessed entrance, leads out onto well-manicured, verdant grounds. Designed by Hellmuth, Obata & Kassabaum, the largest architectural firm in the United States, and completed in 2006, the building houses the courts of Kent County, a collection of mostly working-class towns in central Rhode Island. Given the desultory nature of the business conducted inside, the appealing exterior is disorienting. As one disgruntled local observed in a Google review, "The place looks great while they rob your money in nice suits and bad attitudes."[1]

When I visited the courthouse in the fall of 2019, my purpose was not to investigate architecture or attitudes. I was curious about lawsuits. Usually, when doctors hear the word "lawsuits," our minds immediately turn to our own fears. Personal injury lawyers serving subpoenas for alleged medical malpractice are among the most terrifying figures in medical lore. We share horror stories of these cases and our pet theories about how to ward them off. Some of the cases adjudicated by the courts in this judicial complex were malpractice cases. But I was interested in lawsuits that ran in the other direction—that is, when hospitals sued patients.

I had heard of the practice of hospitals suing patients over unpaid bills years before, but I always thought of it as a rare and widely derided practice, at least at nonprofit hospitals. After all, when Yale New Haven Hospital's (YNHH) penchant for suing patients was splashed across the pages of the *Wall Street Journal* in 2003, had it not spurred such an outcry that the administrators quickly changed their practices? But in recent months I had read of other cases, at both for-profit and nonprofit hospitals, in stories by investigative journalists at ProPublica and elsewhere. While I was visiting my county courthouse, some of my friends in Baltimore were protesting Johns Hopkins Hospital for suing and garnishing the wages of its own low-wage employees when they were unable to pay their hospital bills.

Were such things happening where I lived? I did not think so. I worked at the largest hospitals in the state and had never heard anything about this. But I knew I was largely ignorant of the collection practices of hospitals, including my own. So here I was, walking into the county courthouse and wondering how local lawyers had ended up with such a lavish workplace.

I walked up to the clerk's desk and asked to be directed to the records. Given the beauty of the building, I was surprised when they pointed me to a dated desktop computer in a small, drab room behind their office. After depositing me there, the staff returned to their main task of collecting court fees from the frustrated citizens who came to their desk. To each weary person who came to the window, they had the same question: "How much are you paying today?"

I opened up the search function on the court records database and started typing in hospitals. For some, the records seemed to be fairly sparse, and the hospital almost always seemed to be the defendant. These were malpractice lawsuits. For these hospitals, the few times they were the plaintiff, they were often filing suits against vendors, usually contractors who had not completed a renovation to their liking.

But when I typed in Rhode Island Hospital, the Miriam Hospital, and Newport Hospital, the three facilities where I worked as an emergency medicine resident, the lists of lawsuits were long, and much different from the lists I had seen for other hospitals. In these cases, the hospitals were often plaintiffs, and the defendants were individual patients being sued for overdue bills.

The tactics taken by the hospital to collect from patients seemed aggressive. In 2017, for instance, a lawyer based in the well-off suburb of East Greenwich and representing the Miriam Hospital, an institution with so many donors that their names covered the floors and walls in the foyer, sued a patient for an unpaid bill of $1,157.55, plus an additional $113.21 in court costs. The notice warned that if the patient did not pay, the sum would soon accumulate interest. The patient replied with a plea: "I can only afford to pay $5 per week, due to financial hardship. I get paid twice per month. I am a single mother, with no other income coming into the home and no state assistance." The lawyer relented, but only slightly, accepting her offer to pay $20 per month. To pay off the debt for a single emergency department (ED) visit, she was obligated to continue with this installment plan every month for the next 5 years.[2]

In looking at the records, it was clear that my employer, the nonprofit hospital system Lifespan, took low-income patients to court. When Newport Hospital sued a patient for $2,150.20 plus court costs, he responded that he relied on Social Security disability income to survive. He spent much of this income on medical costs and had precious little to spare. Still, the hospital lawyer insisted on recouping the entire bill, in $25 monthly installments, to be paid over the next 7 years.[3] This is far longer than debt buyers ask people to repay debts; repayment plans at Capio, the nation's largest health care–exclusive debt buyer, are capped at 2 years.[4]

Some defendants responded that the charges were far higher than they would have expected from a brief ED stay. One complained about the care he had received, claiming that he was sent home with an infection, only to return the next day worse than before.[5] Another said he had been assured by the hospital that his test would be completely covered by insurance.[6] But neither sticker shock nor dissatisfaction seemed to sway the court, which almost always sided with the hospitals.

Some of the defendants never responded to the court notices at all. Perhaps they did not see them, or were at a loss as to how to reply, or hoped that the problem would go away. But ignoring the warnings did not prove a good idea, either, as not showing up in court invariably led to a default judgment in favor of the hospital. If these debtors still did not pay after losing their cases in absentia, their wages were garnished.

As I scrolled through these records on the courthouse computer, I was overcome first with surprise, then anger, and then, most of all, shame. These patients had sought medical attention in moments of vulnerability. We, the doctors and nurses and other health care workers, had used all of our training, and all of our effort, to try to allay their pain, to diagnose their ailments, to ensure that any emergent causes of their symptoms were treated promptly. We had not been in the room when the hospital registrar asked for their insurance cards. Almost the only time I checked to see if the patient had insurance was when certain specialists asked me to look, in order to see whether the patient could afford to see one of their supervising physicians, or whether they would have to settle for the resident-run clinic.

Part of the reason I chose emergency medicine as a specialty was that it was the most unadorned, unpretentious, undistracted way to treat patients in distress. Our lineage is in care of the poor; at Rhode Island Hospital, the outpatient department saw patients free of charge for decades before a budgetary crisis brought on by the Great Depression.[7] In the ED, the physicians rarely wear neckties or stylish outfits or even white coats; the risk of getting soaked with blood or stained with vomit is just too high. We almost all wear scrubs, making it difficult for patients to tell the most senior attending physician from the janitor. Most of the doctors have left their white coats at home for so long that they are buried deep in their closets. The hierarchies of medicine have not ossified in the ED as they have elsewhere in the hospital.

The Rhode Island Hospital ED saw more patients than almost any other in New England. It was a gritty place, in appearance and in the attitudes of the people who worked there. Its conditions were more hardscrabble than the wealthier hospitals an hour north in Boston. When the hospital was either full of patients or short of nurses, we struggled to care for people on gurneys that lined the hallways. Most every night, drunk or psychiatrically unstable patients screamed unspeakable obscenities in the triage bay, next to patients being wheeled in with heart attacks and strokes and broken bones. I worried over some of the hospital's shortcomings, but I loved the place. I was particularly proud that the staff treated patients from all walks of life with care and compassion and skill, even if the facilities lacked much luxury.

Although patients often had to wait to be seen, there were no hassles with making an appointment, and no bankers' hours; we were open 24 hours a day, 7 days a week, 365 days a year. We lived by the motto of emergency medicine: "Anyone, anything, anytime." If you woke up with a toothache in the middle of the night, you might be made to sit in the waiting room, but as soon as we finished with the heart attacks and strokes, we would hear your story, examine you carefully, and treat you as best we could. We did not ask for prior authorizations; if you had an emergency, we ordered the appropriate test. If you needed us, we would be there, and the sicker you were, the faster we saw you. I asked about the patient's job and insurance status when it was relevant for diagnosis or management of her condition. If the patient needed help covering the cost of a prescription or needed a voucher for a ride home, I could get help. Our doors were open to all. The ED, I thought, was one of the last bastions of equity, one place in our inegalitarian society where need, and not privilege, got you to the front of the line.

To my horror, as I scrolled, I was finding out that for many patients, the most lasting impact of their visit to the ED was not symptomatic relief or diagnosis but, rather, financial disaster. The gentler my bedside manner, the more I would appear as part of the con to the patient who ended up in a courtroom. They would likely not remember me at all; if they did, I might be one among the many people who had conspired, with the lawyers and judges and collection agencies, to squeeze them for whatever profits I could. Some patients suspected as much. "You guys are all just trying to make a buck off of me," one told me when I advised a chest X-ray. The fact that I was in residency training, making $60,000 a year while working long hours with no control over or knowledge of the billing and collection process was, for him, no excuse. We were all, I now understood, part of the same rapacious machine. Our hospital filled billboards and television ads with promises of just how much we cared, then set our collection lawyers on poor patients; care be damned.

A few former patients kept coming into my head. There was the kind woman who came in with chest pain. When I advised her to stay overnight for further testing and a cardiology consultation, she turned to her husband with a worried face, then asked how much it would cost. I did not know the answer, so I went around the ED asking every other doctor if they knew. They had no idea. I told her I did not know the cost, but insisted that the medically advisable course was to stay the night. She agreed, reluctantly.

I thought, too, of a young man who came in after an opiate overdose. He had nearly died of hypoxia before the paramedics found him and sprayed Narcan up his nose. After arriving in our ED, he immediately said he had to leave. "I'm uninsured! I can't afford to be here!" he yelled. I tried to calm him, assuring him that we did have charity-care. He was not convinced, and his nurse barely had time to find a Narcan kit to send home with him before he stormed out the door.

Finally, I thought of the resigned face of the woman who came in with a painful, widely metastatic cancer, a malignancy she had left festering for 6 months after she had first noticed a mass, bearing the agony at home, alone. What she said she feared most of all were the bills she would leave to her family if she sought treatment.

All these patients had been worried about medical debt, and they had been right to worry. I was in my mid-thirties and had spent almost my entire life in school studying medicine, history, and health policy. But their suspicions about what the hospital would do to them if they could not afford their bills were more accurate than mine.

I have thought since then about what enraged me so much when I learned that my hospital was suing patients. I would like to think that it was empathy for my patients' struggles. But eventually I realized that my view of medicine still had a touch of what sociologist Emile Durkheim called the sacred.[8] That is, I believed it should lie outside the realm of the everyday hurly-burly of market relations, of buying and selling, of the cold, plain logic of the following offer: Your money or your life. The idea that a patient would be hounded for payment after receiving care from me seemed to profane this sacredness, to drag medicine to a place where it did not belong. I was not given to making Biblical references, and had not attended church regularly since college, but I could not help but fear that the money changers had entered the temple. Like the temple in the Gospel of Mark, my hospital had become a den of robbers.[9]

Health care is, at best, what Paul Farmer called "expert mercy," a wonderful admixture of knowledge and caring that manifests what is best in faith traditions and secular humanism.[10] This notion was evident in the example of the Maryland doctors who voted down an attempt to allow wage garnishment of patient-debtors during the nineteenth century, and in the nurses, hospital workers, and patient advocates who organized against hospital lawsuits at YNHH in the twenty-first century.

The fact that my hospital was suing poor patients was, to me, intolerable. But what could I do? Perhaps, I thought, I would form a group of like-minded workers, then meet with the leadership of Lifespan to demand change. I had been involved in similar advocacy efforts in the past, and so often they had come to naught. In college at Harvard, a group of fellow students and I spent months researching the university's practice of charging terrifically high overhead rates on government grants intended for AIDS treatment for Africans. Millions of dollars, we found, were going to pay for things such as cleaning services on Harvard's campus in Cambridge.[11] Was Harvard's multibillion-dollar endowment not sufficient for these expenses? When we presented our research to Harvard's grants administrators, they responded with derision, insinuating we did not know what we were talking about, although they did nothing to disprove our points. One administrator even suggested we wanted to take money from cancer researchers. When we tried to press our case and ask for more meetings, we were met with the kind of polite disregard with which academic administrators learn how to treat student protestors they plan to wait out until graduation day.

I knew I could not stomach walking into the hospital for months while debt collectors filed more lawsuits against my patients—action had to be swift. And while I was not much of a strategy guru, I suspected that given my rather lowly position on medical training's totem pole, surprise would be important. As Sun Tzu advised in *The Art of War*, I would "emerge to their surprise."[12] The C-suite executives would not be allowed to tell me they would look into it. There would be no polite but meaningless discussions. Their actions had, I believed, already breached an essential trust between patients and physicians and should not be allowed to persist.

I knew that at some other institutions, public exposure had led embarrassed executives to reconsider exploitative collection practices. Perhaps I could write an exposé that would have the same effect? At first, I wrote a few impotent tweets, calling out my hospital and its collection agency, Account Recovery Services. After an anemic few likes, I decided the social media route would not do.

So I turned next to drafting an opinion piece. Personal and angry, yet backed by court records and hospital financial reports, I documented the toll taken by aggressive collection practices on my patients. I hoped to shame not only my own institution but also other hospitals that insisted on taking impoverished debtors to court. I mulled the title for a while before coming up with something direct: "Lifespan, Stop Suing My Patients." I did not pull punches. In arguing that the hospital did not need to sue patients to make ends meet, I made note of the chief executive officer's (CEO) salary:

> The average suit seeks less than $2000. While this amount can be debilitating for a working single mom or a person living on disability income, it doesn't make a dent in hospital finances. Assuming Lifespan keeps up its pace of lawsuits against patients for the rest of the year, it will secure roughly $150,000. This sum represents less than one-hundredth of one percent of the hospital's total annual revenue. It is also 14 times less than Timothy Babineau, Lifespan's CEO, made in 2017.[13]

That last sentence was true, but it would soon cause me trouble.

Some of my friends and mentors had been successful in publishing their own pieces in the pages of major national newspapers. My op-ed, on the other hand, received no response from the editorial boards of the *New York Times*, the *Washington Post*, or the *Boston Globe*. Even the *Providence Journal*, the fading daily that covered the town where I worked, passed on it.

I turned, eventually, to *UpriseRI*, a blog run by a crusading progressive journalist named Steve Ahlquist. Ahlquist was ubiquitous at town meetings and small protests around the state. He covered issues that were too frequently ignored by larger press outlets—issues such as environmental degradation and economic hardship. I had learned about the unvarnished realities of life in Rhode Island from his indefatigable journalism. When I sent my piece to Steve, he agreed to publish it. I was grateful that he thought it was worthy of his site, but I worried that it would cause no stir. After all, I wondered, who aside from a few lefty followers of state and local politics even knew his site existed?

The article was published on a cold Thursday morning in September 2019. I did not hear anything of it that morning, as I began a 12-hour shift with our critical-care emergency medical transport team. But that night, while on my last run, transporting an elderly patient with chest pain, I received a text message from one of my residency program directors, asking me to give her a call.

Diligent and funny and self-consciously maternal, this program director's only request of her residents was that we try not to call her cell phone after 1 AM "unless we needed something." She started by saying that she had read my piece and found it powerful and convincing. But, she said, I had upset some people above her at the hospital. She had received a call that evening from one of the system's vice presidents. He insisted that I was incorrect, that Lifespan did not sue patients. He was also upset that I publicly criticized Lifespan and had not first raised my concerns with the relevant people within the organization. By going straight to the press, I had, they claimed, violated a "social media policy" agreement I signed when I started residency. That agreement had asked me to "try to resolve work-related disputes at work . . . by speaking directly with your co-workers, supervisor or other management-level personnel [rather] than by posting complaints in a blog."[14]

In addition, the vice president (VP) said, by noting that I was an employee of Lifespan in my article without clearance from Lifespan's media professionals, I had violated the social media policy again. That policy stated that trainees had to "make it clear you are speaking for yourself and not on behalf of Lifespan." That, I had assumed, was clear enough from the critical tenor of the entire piece. But I had not said the crucial phrase: "The views expressed are my own and do not reflect the views of my employer."[15]

The program director asked me how certain I was of the claims I made in the article. One hospital executive had warned her that if the VP was right and I was incorrect in my claims, I was "at risk of being criticized by Lifespan publicly or more." That sounded like a rather ominous threat to me. I explained that every claim I made in the article had been backed up by court records. These records, I explained, were publicly available and were cited in numerous footnotes in the article.

She supported my decision not to take the piece down. I agreed to ask Ahlquist to remove the mention of my employment at Rhode Island

Hospital from the bio at the end of the article and added the magic words, even though the fact that I worked at Lifespan and that I did not presume to speak for it was clear from the very premise, and title, of the piece.

The VP was not at all satisfied. Despite his busy schedule, he wanted to meet with me personally. My program director arranged to be in the room for the meeting with me, and she made sure that it would be held in her office. "Our turf," she called it.

At this point, I became worried about my job. Losing a residency spot is a big deal, and it could seriously throw a major wrench into my plans for the future. I wanted to continue practicing as a doctor; I just did not want to bankrupt my patients in the process. I fretted about how to stand my ground without losing my job. I spoke with an employment lawyer, although he was not very specific about what I should expect, or what I should say.

My friends in residency were supportive. I received some words of encouragement from one of the consultant physicians when I called to discuss a patient a few days after the article. "I've got a question for you, sir," she began.

That made me nervous. This doctor was known for her no-nonsense demeanor, and I worried that she was about to grill me on some aspect of patient care I had overlooked. But her question was not about the patient. "Are you the one who wrote that piece about the hospital suing patients?"

"Yes, that was me," I answered, not sure what to expect.

"That took some balls," she said.

The day of the meeting, I was nervous. When we sat down, I was taken aback by the VP's tone. He told me he was hurt that I would not come to him first, before criticizing the institution publicly. He said he had worked to create an environment in which people could raise their concerns.

I told him I was heartened to learn that he wanted to hear people's concerns. But, I continued, I had been so shocked by what I saw in the court records that I thought mine was the correct avenue for remedying the problem.

He then insisted that Lifespan did not sue patients. He explained that the hospital once hired a collection agency that sued patients, but when the hospital executives found out about it, they put a stop to it. Aggressive collections did not take place, he assured me, and low-income patients were given discounted or free care.

I knew this was not true. I had seen the court documents that proved these lawsuits were, in fact, occurring. Historians like me have been accused of being almost comically committed to documentary evidence. So I was not going to let this stand. I explained that I had documentation of

Lifespan's recent lawsuits, more than 100 so far that year, including some in the previous 2 weeks. The VP assured me that if Lifespan was actually suing poor patients, he would know, and would be the first to object. I promised him I would send him the court records to prove to him that Lifespan continued to sue patients.

The VP reiterated his disappointment with me, taking the same tone as a father chagrined by a wayward son. Still, I left the meeting relieved. At least I was not fired. I walked down the hall to rejoin our residency conference. Not by coincidence, another executive was, at that very moment, giving a talk on proper use of social media. "Don't surprise your friends," he repeated, like an incantation, a mantra to live by. It was the same advice he gave me in an in-person meeting a few months later. "I thought our patients were our friends," was all I could think to say.

Soon after our meeting, I sent the VP an Excel spreadsheet listing all the lawsuits Lifespan had filed against patients over the past year for unpaid debts. To his credit, the VP replied quickly. He promised to look into the problem.

Three weeks later, he forwarded an email from another Lifespan executive. She explained that Account Recovery Services (ARS), the medical debt collection agency previously contracted by Lifespan, had been suing patients in Lifespan's name, though she had not been aware of it. These cases were "old inventory" representing debts incurred during care delivered between 2 and 4 years earlier. The collection agency had not, she admitted, been "following protocol for screening patients," although she did not state what the protocol was. She said she had confirmed with ARS that it would halt all court filing activity. ARS had been denied access to Lifespan's financial records, so they could not file additional suits. She promised that she would work to dismiss all outstanding cases and would "pull back inventory" from ARS so it could not pursue any more debts on Lifespan's account. "I am very disappointed with the way ARS handled these cases," she lamented. "Please know that this is not the way we want to conduct business with our patients who cannot afford to pay their medical expenses."

I was glad to see this email but skeptical about the executive's attempt to displace responsibility. Was it really possible that no one in the finance department knew about these lawsuits? Was ignorance really an excuse? A quick look at ARS's company website revealed the organization's pride in having "its own legal department staffed with seasoned and experienced collections attorneys." The homepage promised that the 45-year-old company's "legal staff brings decades of experience in debt collections litigation to bear swiftly and efficiently when needed."[16] The image at the top of the website, a stethoscope draped around a judge's gavel, left little to the imagination.[17] The practices of this local agency could scarcely have been better communicated.

In any case, the field of hospital administration was no stranger to collection agencies and their often heavy-handed tactics. After critical media coverage of the collection tactics of YNHH and other hospitals during the early 2000s, administrators throughout the country learned, if they did not already know, that it was up to them to decide whether their third-party collectors could take patients to court, garnish their wages, and foreclose on their homes. As Scott Johnston, director of the Washington office of the Healthcare Financial Management Association, told *Modern Healthcare* in 2005, "Hospitals can stipulate what should be done in their contracts with collection agencies, so there's no reason for an agency to do anything that the hospital wouldn't approve of so long as those guidelines are spelled out."[18]

When I tried to press my case, asking that the hospital zero the balances on lawsuit judgments already rendered, as many other hospital systems had done, I received no response. Still, I was gratified to learn that the hospital had stopped the worst of its tactics. When I checked the district court records online in subsequent months, it appeared Lifespan executives had kept their word. I did not see any further lawsuits against patients. I could sleep a little better at night.

Still, the restricted scope of these changes shows the limits of my choice of protest. At YNHH, a large coalition of unions and community groups organized a sustained effort to change policies at that medical center and, within a year, across the state. Their work spurred national awareness that, for a time, put hospital collection on the national policy agenda. YNHH's policies were much more aggressive than Rhode Island Hospital's, and its executives much more intransigent, yet they eventually caved to pressure. The power of this sustained organizing proved greater than my much smaller act.

In fact, as of August 2022, Rhode Island had some of the most regressive medical debt laws in the country. Hospitals were not required to offer payment plans prior to sending bills to collections. State law set no minimum amount of time a collector had to wait before filing suit. No restrictions existed on bank executions, wage garnishments, home foreclosures, or body attachments. According to Innovation for Justice, a collaboration between researchers at the University of Arizona and the University of Utah, Rhode Island ranked 46 out of 50 states for medical debt consumer protection policy. The only other states to score as poorly were West Virginia, Texas, South Carolina, and Tennessee. The best score went to Maryland, which had passed a series of protections against aggressive medical debt collection in 2020 and 2021 (see Chapter 5).[19] Even with these differences in state laws, everywhere in the country patients remained vulnerable to predation and financial ruin when they sought care. Medicine was no refuge for the sick, the hospital no haven. The work of providing a just place for the sick to find care and respite remained unfinished.

NOTES

INTRODUCTION

1. Wes Allison, "Working Cure," *Richmond Times-Dispatch*, March 20, 1995.
2. Allison, "Working Cure."
3. Corey Stone, *Shining a Light on the Consumer Debt Industry*, Senate Subcommittee on Financial Institutions and Consumer Protection of the Committee on Banking, Housing and Urban Affairs, July 17, 2013, 4.
4. "Bad Debt Exceeds $10M at a Third of Organizations, But Lack of Confidence Exists in How Much Is Recoverable," Sage Growth Partners, June 19, 2018.
5. Cheryl Cooper, "The Debt Collection Market and Policy Issues," Congressional Research Service Report R46477, June 22, 2021.
6. Farah Hashim et al., "Characteristics of US Hospitals Using Extraordinary Collections Actions Against Patients for Unpaid Medical Bills: A Cross-Sectional Study," *BMJ Open* 12 (20220): e060501.
7. Some hospital officials say they rarely sue patients, or no longer sue patients, even if their hospital policies allow for it. See Noam Levey, "Investigation: Many US Hospitals Sue Patients for Debts or Threaten Their Credit," NPR, December 21, 2022.
8. Noam Levey, "Sick and Struggling to Pay, 100 Million People in the U.S. Live with Medical Debt," NPR, June 16, 2022.
9. Raymond Kluender et al., "Medical Debt in the US, 2009–2020," *Journal of the American Medical Association* 326, no. 3 (2021): 250–56.
10. See Elizabeth Warren and Amelia Warren Tyagi, *The Two-Income Trap: Why Middle-Class Parents Are Going Broke* (New York: Basic Books, 2004); Teresa Sullivan, Jay Lawrence Westbrook, and Elizabeth Warren, *As We Forgive Our Debtors: Bankruptcy and Consumer Credit in America* (Fairless Hills, PA: Beard Books, 1999).
11. David Graeber, *Debt: The First 5,000 Years* (New York: Melville House, 2011), 5.
12. Consumer Financial Protection Bureau, "Medical Debt Burden in the United States," March 2022.
13. "1 in 10 Adults Owe Medical Debt, with Millions Owing More Than $10,000," Kaiser Family Foundation, March 10, 2022, https://www.kff.org/health-costs/press-release/1-in-10-adults-owe-medical-debt-with-millions-owing-more-than-10000/#:~:text=A%20new%20KFF%20analysis%20of,who%20owe%20more%20than%20%2410%2C000.
14. Kluender et al., "Medical Debt in the US," 254.
15. Kluender et al., "Medical Debt in the US," 254.

16. Levey, "Sick and Struggling to Pay."
17. Robert Saywell et al., "Hospital and Patient Characteristics of Uncompensated Hospital Care: Policy Implications," *Journal of Health Politics, Policy and Law* 14, no. 2 (1989): 287–307; Joel Weissman et al., "Bad Debt and Free Care in Massachusetts Hospitals," *Health Affairs* 11, no. 2 (1992): 148–61.
18. Levey, "Sick and Struggling to Pay."
19. Yang Wang et al., "COVID-19 and Hospital Financial Viability in the US," *JAMA Health Forum* 3, no. 5 (2022): e221018; see also Levey, "Sick and Struggling to Pay."
20. Rozanne Anderson, "Powering up the Rev Cycle—Hot Topics for Healthcare Providers," *InsideARM*, November 22, 2017.
21. Crystal Ewing, "Hospitals Seek Out New Ways to Reduce Bad Debt, Focus on Self-Pay Patients," *Becker's Hospital Review*, November 14, 2017.
22. M. P. Pell, "Patients in Arrears Face Collectors: Agencies Buy up Delinquent Accounts," *Atlanta Journal-Constitution*, June 5, 2011.
23. Will Bruhn et al., "Prevalence and Characteristics of Virginia Hospitals Suing Patients and Garnishing Wages for Unpaid Medical Bills," *Journal of the American Medical Association* 322, no. 7 (2019): 691–92.
24. Selena Simmons-Duffin, "When Hospitals Sue for Unpaid Bills, It Can Be 'Ruinous' for Patients," NPR, June 25, 2019.
25. Tara Bannow, "Few Hospitals Aggressively Sue Patients to Pay Bills," *Modern Healthcare*, October 5, 2019.
26. Marty Makary, *The Price We Pay: What Broke American Healthcare and How to Fix It* (New York: Bloomsbury, 2019), 57.
27. Ashley Kirzinger et al., "Data Note: Americans' Challenges with Health Care Costs." Kaiser Family Foundation, June 11, 2019, https://www.kff.org/health-costs/issue-brief/data-note-americans-challenges-health-care-costs/view/footnotes.
28. David Himmelstein et al., "Prevalence and Risk Factors for Medical Debt and Subsequent Changes in Social Determinants of Health in the US," *JAMA Network Open* 5, no. 9 (2022): e2231898.
29. "Americans' Views of Healthcare Costs, Coverage and Policy," Westhealth Institute, 2018, https://www.norc.org/PDFs/WHI%20Healthcare%20Costs%20Coverage%20and%20Policy/WHI%20Healthcare%20Costs%20Coverage%20and%20Policy%20Issue%20Brief.pdf.
30. Andre Perry, Carl Romer, and Nana Adjeiwaa-Manu, "The Racial Implications of Medical Debt: How Moving Toward Universal Health Care and Other Reforms Can Address Them," Brookings Institute, October 5, 2021.
31. Chi Chi Wu, "Medical Debt," *Clearinghouse Review Journal of Poverty Law and Policy* 39, nos. 7–8 (2005): 465–85, 467.
32. Beatrix Hoffman, "Restraining the Health Care Consumer: Deductibles and Copayments in U.S. Health Insurance," *Social Science History* 30, no. 4 (2006): 501–28, 520.
33. Michelle Doty et al., "Seeing Red: Americans Driven into Debt by Medical Bills," The Commonwealth Fund, August 2005.
34. This study found that credit card debt was the only other kind of consumer debt with a strong association with forgone care: Lucie Kalousova and Sarah Burgard, "Debt and Foregone Medical Care," *Journal of Health and Social Behavior* 54, no. 2 (2013): 204–20.

35. Alyce Adams et al., "The Impact of Financial Assistance Programs on Health Care Utilization," National Bureau of Economic Research, Working Paper 29227, August 31, 2021.
36. Simmons-Duffin, "When Hospitals Sue."
37. Kelly Gooch, "70% of Americans Trust Their Physicians, 22% Trust Hospital Execs, Survey Finds," *Becker's Hospital Review*, August 10, 2021.
38. American Hospital Association, "Fast Facts on US Hospitals, 2022," 2022, https://www.aha.org/system/files/media/file/2022/01/fast-facts-on-US-hospitals-2022.pdf.
39. Sixty-three percent of people in the top 5 percent of annual medical spending experienced a hospitalization in that year. See Carlos Dobkin et al., "Myth and Measurement: The Case of Medical Bankruptcies," *New England Journal of Medicine* 378, no. 12 (2018): 1076–78.
40. George Orwell, "Politics and the English Language," in *A Collection of Essays* (Orlando, FL: Harvest, 1981), 167.
41. See, for instance, Robert Goff and Jerry Ashton, *The Patient, the Doctor, the Bill Collector: A Medical Debt Survival Guide* (Kauai, HI: Hoku House, 2016); Marshall Allen, *Never Pay the First Bill: And Other Ways to Fight the Health Care System and Win* (New York: Portfolio, 2021); Strike Debt, *The Debt Resistors' Operations Manual*, September 2012.
42. Raj Tek Sehgal and Paul Gorman, "Internal Medicine Physicians' Knowledge of Health Care Charges," *Journal of Graduate Medical Education* 3, no. 2 (2011): 182–87.

CHAPTER 1

1. Peter Coleman, *Debtors and Creditors in America: Insolvency, Imprisonment for Debt, and Bankruptcy, 1607–1900* (Fairless Hills, PA: Beard Books, 1999), 193–94.
2. US Department of Health, Education, and Welfare, *Medical Care in Transition, Volume 2* (Washington, DC: Government Printing Office, 1964), 266.
3. Leonard Richards, *Shays Rebellion: The American Revolution's Final Battle* (Philadelphia: University of Pennsylvania Press, 2003).
4. Thomas Bard Jones, "Legacy of Change: The Panic of 1819 and Debtor Relief Legislation in the Western States" (PhD diss., Cornell University, 1968), ProQuest Dissertations.
5. Gustav Peebles, "Washing Away the Sins of Debt: The Nineteenth-Century Eradication of the Debtors' Prison," *Comparative Studies in Society and History* 55, no. 3 (2013): 702.
6. Harlow Giles Unger, *John Quincy Adams* (New York: Hachette, 2012), 246.
7. Andrew Jackson, "Third Annual Message, December 6, 1831," The American Presidency Project (n.d.), https://www.presidency.ucsb.edu/documents/third-annual-message-3.
8. *A Pound of Flesh: The Criminalization of Private Debt*, American Civil Liberties Union, 2018, 4.
9. "A Brief History of Debt Collection and Its Regulation in the United States," National Consumer Law Center Digital Library, https://library.nclc.org.
10. Tamara Plaikins Thornton, "'A Great Machine' or a 'Beast of Prey': A Boston Corporation and Its Rural Debtors in an Age of Capitalist Transformation," *Journal of the Early American Republic* 27, no. 4 (2007): 567–97.
11. "*New England Journal of Medicine and Surgery, XIV*, 1825, 53–54," quoted in George Rosen, *Fees and Fee Bills: Some Economic Aspects of Medical Practice in Nineteenth Century America* (Baltimore: Johns Hopkins University Press, 1946), 6–7.

12. Rosen, *Fees and Fee Bills*, 2–15.
13. Rosen, *Fees and Fee Bills*, 50.
14. Rosen, *Fees and Fee Bills*, 13.
15. Rosen, *Fees and Fee Bills*, 36.
16. Rosen, *Fees and Fee Bills*, 45–46.
17. "F.L.J.," in the *St. Louis Medical and Surgical Journal* (year unknown), quoted in Taylor, *The Physician as a Business Man*, 99.
18. Taylor, *The Physician as a Business Man*, 99–108.
19. Taylor, *The Physician as a Business Man*, 99–108.
20. Brian Jones, *Healing Rhode Island: The Story of Rhode Island Hospital, 1863–2013* (East Providence, RI: Signature Printing, 2013), 16.
21. Charles Rosenberg, *The Care of Strangers: The Rise of America's Hospital System* (New York: Basic Books, 1987), 34–36.
22. David Rosner, *A Once Charitable Enterprise: Hospitals and Health Care in Brooklyn and New York, 1885–1915* (New York: Cambridge University Press, 1982).
23. Rosner, *A Once Charitable Enterprise*, 108–11.
24. Aniel Webster Cathell, *The Physician Himself from Graduation to Old Age* (Philadelphia: Davis, 1925), 292, quoted in Melissa Jacoby and Mirya Holman, "Managing Medical Bills on the Brink of Bankruptcy," *Yale Journal of Health Policy, Law and Ethics* 10, no. 2 (2010): 240.
25. *Transactions of the Medical and Chirurgical Faculty of the State of Maryland, 91st Annual Session, Held at Baltimore, Md. April 1889* (Baltimore: Press of Isaac Friedenwald, 1889), 16.
26. Rosemary Stevens, *In Sickness and in Wealth: American Hospitals in the Twentieth Century* (Baltimore: Johns Hopkins University Press, 1999), 26–27, 42.
27. Nancy Tomes, *Remaking the American Patient: How Madison Avenue and Modern Medicine Turned Patients into Consumers* (Chapel Hill: University of North Carolina Press, 2016), 68.
28. George F. Shrady, "A Propagator of Pauperism: The Dispensary," *The Forum* 23 (June 1897): 425, quoted in Paul Starr, *The Social Transformation of American Medicine: The Rise of a Sovereign Profession and the Making of a Vast Industry* (New York: Basic Books, 1982), 182.
29. "Worried by Debt, He Tries Suicide," *Atlanta Journal-Constitution*, October 10, 1912.
30. Beatrix Hoffman, *Health Care for Some: Rights and Rationing in the United States Since 1930* (Chicago: University of Chicago Press, 2012), 63–64.
31. Hoffman, *Health Care for Some*, 19.
32. Hoffman, *Health Care for Some*, 86.
33. Hoffman, *Health Care for Some*.
34. Hoffman, *Health Care for Some*, 34.
35. Stevens, *In Sickness and in Wealth*, 146. The term dunning is, by some accounts, derived from the seventeenth-century English term meaning to demand payment for a debt. See Kitty O. Locker, "'Sir, This Will Never Do': Model Dunning Letters, 1592–1873," *Journal of Business Communication* 22, no. 2 (1973): 39–45.
36. Stevens, *In Sickness and in Wealth*, 265.
37. Stevens, *In Sickness and in Wealth*, 267.
38. Stevens, *In Sickness and in Wealth*, 269.
39. Lyndon Johnson, "Remarks with President Truman at the Signing in Independence of the Medicare Bill, July 30, 1965," The American Presidency

Project, n.d., https://www.presidency.ucsb.edu/documents/remarks-with-presid ent-truman-the-signing-independence-the-medicare-bill.

40. A regression discontinuity analysis found that "Medicare reduced the annual probability of large medical collections, above $1,000, by 0.31 percentage points, a 19 percent reduction relative to the probability for those aged 60–64"; see Kyle Caswell and John Goddeeris, "Does Medicare Reduce Medical Debt?," *American Journal of Health Economics* 6, no. 1 (Winter 2020).

41. *Parker v City of Highland Park, Michigan*, 404 Mich. 183 (Supreme Court of Michigan, 1978). This case ended "charitable immunity," a liability protection against negligence that was given to voluntary hospitals in some states until the 1960s and to some local government hospitals until this decision. See Stevens, *In Sickness and in Wealth*, 41.

42. Gabriel Winant, *The Next Shift; The Fall of Industry and the Rise of Health Care in Rust Belt America* (Boston: Harvard University Press, 2021), 148.

43. Louis Hyman, *Debtor Nation: The History of America in Red Ink* (Princeton, NJ: Princeton University Press, 2011), 15–16.

44. Hyman, *Debtor Nation*, 83–84.

45. Leon Henderson, *The Use of Small Loans for Medical Expenses* (Washington, DC: Committee on the Costs of Medical Care, 1930), 9.

46. Olin W. Anderson, "National Consumer Survey of Medical Costs and Voluntary Health Insurance," in *Health Inquiry: Hearings Before the Committee on Interstate and Foreign Commerce, House of Representatives* (Washington, DC: Government Printing Office, 1954).

47. John Frechtling and Irving Schweiger, "1952 Survey of Consumer Finances, Part III: Income, Selected Investments and Short-Term Debt of Consumers," *Federal Reserve Bulletin* (September 1952): 974–1001, https://fraser.stlouisfed.org/title/ federal-reserve-bulletin-62/september-1952-21213.

48. Internal Revenue Service, Rev. Rul. 56–185, 1956–1 C.B. 202, 1956, https:// www.irs.gov/pub/irs-tege/rr56-185.pdf. Also see Mark Everson, Commissioner, Internal Revenue Service, quoted in US House of Representatives Committee on Ways and Means, *The Tax-Exempt Hospital Sector* (Washington, DC: Government Printing Office, 2005), 12.

49. John Colombo, quoted in *The Tax-Exempt Hospital Sector*, 87.

50. Colombo, quoted in *The Tax-Exempt Hospital Sector*, 7.

51. Also see Everson, quoted in *The Tax-Exempt Hospital Sector*, 12.

52. Robert Bromberg, "The Charitable Hospital," *Catholic University Law Review* 20, no. 2 (1970): 243.

53. Bromberg, "The Charitable Hospital," 258.

54. Ge Bai and David Hyman, "Tax Exemptions for Nonprofit Hospitals: It's Time Taxpayers Get Their Money's Worth," *STATNews*, April 5, 2021. Also see Colombo, quoted in *The Tax-Exempt Hospital Sector*, 88.

55. Robert Bromberg, "Financing Health Care and the Effect of the Tax Law," *Law and Contemporary Problems* 39, no. 4 (1975): 156–82.

56. Edward M. Kennedy, *In Critical Condition: The Crisis in America's Health Care* (New York: Simon & Schuster, 1971), 179.

57. Daniel Schorr, *Don't Get Sick in America* (Chicago: Aurora Publishers, 1970), 45.

58. Schorr, *Don't Get Sick in America*, 39.

59. Schorr, *Don't Get Sick in America*, 34.

60. "Hijacker Is Slain; Said Deep in Debt over Medical Bills," *The Washington Post*, January 28, 1972.

61. "Hijacker Is Slain."

62. Teresa Sullivan, Jay Lawrence Westbrook, and Elizabeth Warren, *As We Forgive Our Debtors: Bankruptcy and Consumer Credit in America* (Fairless Hills, PA: Beard Books, 1999), 168.

63. Elizabeth Warren and Amelia Warren Tyagi, *The Two-Income Trap: Why Middle-Class Parents Are Going Broke* (New York: Basic Books, 2004).

CHAPTER 2

1. Michael Katz, *The Price of Citizenship: Redefining the American Welfare State* (Philadelphia: University of Pennsylvania Press, 2008).

2. Maureen Santini, "Mondale Says Reagan 'Out of Step with America,'" Associated Press, August 14, 1980.

3. "Social Welfare Under Reagan," CQ Press, March 9, 1984.

4. Ralph Regula, "National Policy and the Medically Uninsured," *Inquiry* 24, no. 1 (1987): 48–56.

5. This was the 1982 Tax Equity and Fiscal Responsibility Act (TEFRA). For more on the politics of this moment, see Jonathan Oberlander, *The Political Life of Medicaid* (Chicago: University of Chicago Press, 2003), 122–24.

6. Regula, "National Policy," 48–56.

7. Helen Darling, "The Role of the Federal Government in Assuring Access to Health Care," *Inquiry* 23, no. 3 (1986): 286–96.

8. John Klemm, "Medicaid Spending: A Brief History," *Health Care Financing Review* 22, no. 1 (2000): 105–12.

9. "Disproportionate Share Hospital Payments," Medicaid and CHIP Payment and Access Commission, https://www.macpac.gov/subtopic/disproportionate-share-hospital-payments/#:~:text=Medicaid%20disproportionate%20share%20hospital%20(DSH,stability%20of%20safety%2Dnet%20hospitals.

10. Oberlander, *The Political Life of Medicaid*, 125.

11. R. Paul Duncan and Kerry Kilpatrick, "Unresolved Hospital Charges in Florida," *Health Affairs* 6, no. 1 (1987): 159–60.

12. David Cutler, "Cost Shifting or Cost Cutting? The Incidence of Reductions in Medicare Payments," in *Tax Policy and the Economy*, vol. 12, ed. James Poterba (Cambridge, MA: MIT Press, 1998), 1–28, http://www.nber.org/chapters/c10911. Also see Donald Cohodes, "America: The Home of the Free, the Land of the Uninsured," *Inquiry* 23 (1986): 227–35.

13. David Cutler et al., "How Does Managed Care Do It?," *Rand Journal of Economics* 31, no. 3 (2000): 526–48.

14. David Cutler, "Equality, Efficiency, and Market Fundamentals: The Dynamics of International Medical Reform," *Journal of Economic Literature* 40, no. 3 (2002): 900.

15. Ronald Reagan, "The President's News Conference," November 10, 1981, The Reagan Library Archives Online, https://www.reaganlibrary.gov/archives/speech/presidents-news-conference.

16. The cost of uncompensated care (not charges) increased from $2.8 billion to $5.7 billion during this time. See Cohodes, "America."

17. Douglas Sherlock, "Indigent Care in Rational Markets," *Inquiry* 23, no. 3 (1986): 261–67.

18. Frederic Michas, "Number of Hospitals in the U.S., 1975–2019," *Statista*, February 9, 2021. Another chart that shows a similar decline is found in Leiyu

Shi and Douglas Singh, *Delivering Health Care in America: A Systems Approach*, 7th ed. (Burlington, MA: Jones & Bartlett, 2017), Figure 8.2, 356.

19. Sherlock, "Indigent Care in Rational Markets," 261–67.
20. David Clark, "Profits, Publicity Fuel Trend Toward Marketing of Health-Care Services," *Christian Science Monitor*, December 5, 1984. For a more up-to-date account of the kinds of hospitals in each state, see Kaiser Family Foundation, "Hospital by Ownership Type: 2020," https://www.kff.org/other/state-indica tor/hospitals-by-ownership/?currentTimeframe=0&sortModel=%7B%22co lId%22:%22Location%22,%22sort%22:%22asc%22%7D.
21. Regula, "National Policy," 55.
22. Beatrix Hoffman, "Emergency Rooms: The Reluctant Safety Net," in *History and Health Policy in the United States: Putting the Past Back In*, eds. Rosemary Stevens, Charles Rosenberg, and Lawton Burns (New Brunswick: Rutgers University Press, 2006), 250–72.
23. David Himmelstein et al., "Patient Transfers: Medical Practices as Social Triage," *American Journal of Public Health* 74, no. 5 (1984): 494–97.
24. Beatrix Hoffman, *Health Care for Some* (Chicago: University of Chicago Press).
25. Sandra Friedland, "Hospitals Worried About Fund for Poor," *New York Times*, December 23, 1990.
26. Suzanne Mulstein, "The Uninsured and the Financing of Uncompensated Care: Scope, Costs and Policy Options," *Inquiry* 21, no. 3 (1984): 214–29. See also Judith Nemes, "Hospitals Put Teeth into Efforts to Collect Bad Debt," *Modern Healthcare* 21, no. 24 (1991): 41–50.
27. Nemes, "Hospitals Put Teeth into Efforts."
28. Jason Callicoat and David Rumbach, "Medical Debt Problem Requires Creative Thinking," *South Bend Tribune*, July 2, 2001.
29. Stephen Alexander Magnus, "Agency Implications of Debt in Not-for-Profit Hospitals" (PhD. diss., University of Michigan, 2002), 47–50.
30. Nemes, "Hospitals Put Teeth into Efforts," 41–50.
31. Robert Seifert, "The Demand Side of Financial Exploitation: The Case of Medical Debt," *Housing Policy Debate* 15, no. 3 (2010): 795.
32. Gerard Anderson, "Testimony Before House of Representatives," in *US House of Representatives Committee on Energy and Commerce: Review of Hospital Billing and Collection Practices* (Washington, DC: Government Printing Office, 2004), 18–21.
33. Anderson, "Testimony."
34. Gerard Anderson, "From 'Soak the Rich' to 'Soak the Poor': Recent Trends in Hospital Pricing," *Health Affairs* 26, no. 3 (2007): 780–89.
35. Gerard Anderson explained in 2004 that "hospitals routinely quantify the amount of bad debt and charity care they provide. . . . By valuing bad debt and charity care at full charges, these numbers vastly overestimate the amount of bad debt and charity care the hospital actually provides." In personal correspondence in 2022, Anderson explained that hospitals were forced to change their practice, and value charity care using costs rather than charges, only when the IRS set more stringent reporting requirements in 2010. Anderson, "Testimony."
36. The Access Project, *The Consequences of Medical Debt: Evidence from Three Communities*, February 2003.
37. In 2003, Ray Lefton, a dentist-cum-accountant who served as the chief financial officer of Temple University's cash-strapped Northeastern Hospital in an impoverished Black neighborhood in Philadelphia, eagerly explained

in *Healthcare Financial Management* how he was building a new room in the emergency department to "aggressively" collect payment from uninsured patients after discharge. Lefton explained this was Plan B—his original idea had been abandoned due to "public-relations concerns." His favorite plan would have required emergency department patients to fork over "some minimum payment" after their initial triage but "before we will complete treatment." Ray Lefton, "What's It Worth? Cost Shifting, a Practice That Can Often Result in Significant Financial Burden on Self-Pay Patients, Is Leading to Greater Scrutiny of Hospital Charging Practices," *Healthcare Financial Management* 57, no. 12 (2003): 60.

38. Kim Crompton, "Spokane Hospitals Soft-Pedal Debt Collections," *Spokane Journal of Business* 7, no. 19 (October 1992): B3.
39. Nemes, "Hospitals Put Teeth into Efforts," 41.
40. Cohodes, "America," 232.
41. Personal interview with Ruth Lande, August 22, 2022.
42. Lisa Scott, "Firm Offers to Sell Bad Debt to Highest Bidder," *Modern Healthcare*, February 8, 1993.
43. Crompton, "Spokane Hospitals."
44. Stone, "Firm Offers to Sell Bad Debt," 7.
45. Chulho Christopher Lee, "The Financial Impacts of Bad Debt in the Healthcare Industry: A Multivariate Statistical Analysis" (PhD diss., St. Louis University, 1996).
46. Katherine Acosta, "Surviving the American Health Care System: Experiences and Strategies of Uninsured Women" (PhD diss., University of Nebraska, 2003).
47. Thomas O'Toole et al., "Full Disclosure of Financial Costs and Options to Patients: The Roles of Race, Age, Health Insurance, and Usual Source for Care," *Journal of Healthcare for the Poor and Underserved* 15, no. 1 (2004): 52–62.
48. Lisa Duchon et al., "Security Matters: How Instability in Health Insurance Puts U.S. Workers at Risk," *The Commonwealth Fund*, December 2001, vii, 9–12.
49. Caitlin Devitt, "Taking the Pulse on Healthcare Collections: How Will Healthcare Collections Change as Reform Plans Sweep the Country?," *Collections & Credit Risk* 12, no. 9 (2007): 18.
50. Caitlin Devitt, "A Debt Rx for Healthcare: Hospitals Are Dealing with More and More Bad Debt, Trying to Figure out Whether and When They Should Sell and What Role Collection Should Pay," *Collections and Credit Risk* 11, no. 10 (2006): 34.
51. Scott, "Firm Offers to Sell Bad Debt," 34.
52. Scott, "Firm Offers to Sell Bad Debt," 34.
53. Scott, "Firm Offers to Sell Bad Debt," 34.
54. Allan Sloan, "The SEC vs Steven Hoffenberg: A Case of Leaning Fortunes at Towers Financial?," *Washington Post*, February 16, 1993.
55. "Jeffrey Epsteins's Mentor—Who Once Ran a Ponzi Scheme—Was Found Dead. He Was 77," Associated Press, August 26, 2022.
56. Richard Gunderman, "Medicine and the Pursuit of Wealth," *Hastings Center Report* 28, no. 1 (1998): 9.
57. Caitlin Devitt, "Medical Debt Heavy Hitters," *Collections & Credit Risk* 12, no. 5 (May 2007): 48–55.
58. "Stirrings in Medical Debt," *Collections & Credit Risk* 5, no. 7 (July 2000), 18.
59. Tom Murphy, "Health Care Company Grows by Piling up Debt: After Six Years, Senex Services Corp. Expands Its Collection Business in a Field That Is Ripe for Growth," *Indianapolis Business Journal* 24, no. 53 (2004), 9..

60. Encore Capital Group, "Business Update: September–October 2005," https://www.sec.gov/Archives/edgar/data/1084961/000119312505191671/dex991.htm.
61. MP Pell, "Patients in Arrears Face Collectors: Agencies Buy Up Delinquent Accounts," *The Atlanta Journal-Constitution*, June 5, 2011, B1.
62. Devitt, "A Debt Rx for Healthcare," 34.
63. Devitt, "A Debt Rx for Healthcare," 34.
64. Devitt, "Taking the Pulse on Healthcare Collections."
65. Janice Boyd, "The Debt Buying Market Comes of Age," *Collector* 86, no. 12 (2021): 40–41.
66. Cynthia Wilson, "Health Care Receivables Pose More Challenges Than Opportunities for Big Debt Collectors," *Inside ARM*, March 7, 2011.
67. Andrea Murphy, "America's Largest Private Companies: Cargill Is Back at No. 1," *Forbes*, November 23, 2021.
68. Devitt, "Medical Debt Heavy Hitters," 54.
69. "Encore Capital Group Enters Healthcare Debt Market with a Purchase of $300 Million Portfolio and Hiring of General Manager for Medical Business," Encore Capital Group, September 8, 2005.
70. Encore Capital Group, "Business Update, September–October 2005."
71. See Chapter 2 of Jake Halpern, *Bad Paper: Inside the Secret World of Debt Collectors* (New York: Picador, 2015).
72. Vivian Marino, "Debt Collectors Thrive as Borrowers Binge," *Las Vegas Review*, April 15, 1996.
73. Encore Capital Group, "Business Update: September—October 2005."
74. Gregory Potts, "Surprising Rewards in Debt Collection," *Journal Record* (Oklahoma City), September 13, 1999.
75. Marino, "Debt Collectors Thrive."
76. Albert Crenshaw, "Bill Collectors' Abusive Tactics Under Scrutiny," *Washington Post*, September 13, 1992.
77. Acosta, "Surviving the American Health Care System," 151–52.
78. Seifert, "The Demand Side," 795.
79. Melissa Jacoby, "Testimony Before Hearing of House Committee on Energy and Commerce," in *US House of Representatives Committee on Energy and Commerce: Review of Hospital Billing and Collections Practices* (Washington, DC: Government Printing Office, 2004), 27.
80. Consumer Financial Protection Bureau, "Medical Debt Burden in the United States," February 2022.
81. Ray Lefton, "Developing Organizational Charity-Care Policies and Procedures," *Healthcare Financial Management* 52 (April 2002): 54–55.
82. Representative Jan Schakowsky, "Testimony Before Hearing of House Committee on Energy and Commerce," in *US House of Representatives Committee on Energy and Commerce: Review of Hospital Billing Collections and Practices* (Washington, DC: Government Printing Office, 2004), 7.
83. Dennis O'Brien, "Hospitals Sue to Collect from Uninsured Patients," *Baltimore Sun*, August 15, 1993.
84. David Graeber, *Debt: The First 5,000 Years* (New York: Melville House, 2011), 13.
85. "Allowing Low-Income Hospital Patients to Work off Their Hospital Bills," *Healthcare PR and Marketing News* 7, no. 5 (March 1998).
86. "Allowing Low-Income Hospital Patients to Work."

CHAPTER 3

1. See, for instance, the "About Us" section of the debt collection firm ARS National Services, https://www.arsnational.com (accessed July 11, 2022).
2. David Reid, *The Debt Buying Industry*, White Paper of the Receivables Management Association International, 2016, 2, https://rmaintl.org/wp-content/uploads/2019/01/White-Paper-The-Debt-Buying-Industry_Executive_Summary.pdf
3. Reid, *The Debt Buying Industry*, 2.
4. *The Impact of Third-Party Debt Collection on the National and State Economies*, Ernst & Young, January 2012, https://www.creditandcollectionnews.com/uploads/The%20Impact%20of%203rd%20Party%20Debt%20Collection%20on%20the%20National%20and%20State%20Economies.pdf.
5. Jake Halpern, *Bad Paper: Inside the Secret World of Debt Collectors* (New York: Picador, 2015).
6. Consumer Financial Protection Bureau, "Study of Third-Party Debt Collection Operations," July 2016, https://www.consumerfinance.gov/data-research/research-reports/study-third-party-debt-collection-operations.
7. "Debt Collection Agencies in the US, Number of Businesses 2005–2008," IBIS World, June 28, 2022, https://www.ibisworld.com/industry-statistics/number-of-businesses/debt-collection-agencies-united-states.
8. Consumer Financial Protection Bureau, "Study of Third-Party Debt Collection Operations."
9. Consumer Financial Protection Bureau, "Study of Third-Party Debt Collection Operations."
10. Consumer Financial Protection Bureau, "Study of Third-Party Debt Collection Operations."
11. ACA International, "Diversity in the Collections Industry: Examining the Demographics of Collection Agents," 2022, https://www.acainternational.org/wp-content/uploads/2022/08/Diversity-in-the-Collections-Industry-2022-FinalACA.pdf
12. Larry Lewis, "Big Collections from Little Debts Have a Montco Firm Growing," *Philadelphia Inquirer*, January 16, 1992.
13. Jay Finegan, "48 Hours with the King of Cold Calls," *Inc.*, June 1991.
14. "Chuck Piola," Catholic Speakers Organization Profiles, accessed January 14, 2023, https://catholicspeakers.com/profiles/chuck-piola.
15. Consumer Financial Protection Bureau, "Study of Third-Party Debt Collection Operations," 27.
16. Lewis, "Big Collections."
17. Lewis, "Big Collections."
18. Chuck Piola, *Going in Cold: How to Turn Strangers into Clients and Get Rich Doing It* (Washington, DC: Folger Ross, 2005), 12.
19. Finegan, "48 Hours."
20. Lewis, "Big Collections."
21. Piola, *Going in Cold*, 11.
22. Joseph DiStefano, "Despite Criticism, Debt Collector Keeps Expanding," *Philadelphia Inquirer*, July 21, 2013.
23. Finegan, "48 Hours."
24. Andrea Ahles, "Fort Washington, PA, Collection Agency Finds Profit in Others' Debt," *Philadelphia Inquirer*, December 21, 1998.

25. Prabha Natarajan, "No Grass Under These Young Feet: Three CEOs Strike Gold Before 40," *Philadelphia Business Journal*, August 2, 1999.
26. NCO Group, Inc., Encyclopedia.com, https://www.encyclopedia.com/books/politics-and-business-magazines/nco-group-inc.
27. "Profile—NCO Group, Inc. (NasdaqNM: NCOG)," Yahoo Finance, accessed January 14, 2023, https://pages.cs.wisc.edu/~anhai/wisc-si-archive/data/company_profiles/yahoo/instances/company-index/Services/Business_Services/instances/http:%5E%5Ebiz.yahoo.com%5Ep%5En%5Encog.html.
28. Caitlin Devitt, "Medical Debt Heavy Hitters," *Collections & Credit Risk* 12, no. 5 (2007): 55.
29. Devitt, "Medical Debt Heavy Hitters," 55.
30. "Transworld Systems Signs Agreement with AMA to Provide Accounts Receivable Management Solutions to Member Physicians," InsideARM, March 7, 2011.
31. NCO Group, Inc., Encyclopedia.com.
32. "Q3 2004 NCO Group Earnings Conference Call," Fair Disclosure Wire, November 2, 2004, accessed via Gale OneFile: Business.
33. "Q1 2005 NCO Group Earnings Conference Call," Fair Disclosure Wire, May 3, 2005, accessed via Gale OneFile: Business.
34. "NCO Portfolio, Medclr in Agreement to Purchase $500 Million in Medical Receivables," InsideARM, September 12, 2006.
35. Devitt, "Medical Debt Heavy Hitters," 54.
36. Jeff Blumenthal, "New CEO to Take over at Debt Collector NCO," *Philadelphia Business Journal*, March 21, 2011.
37. "Fifteen Distinguished Alumni Elected to the Drexel 100," *The Drexel 100 Newsletter,* Drexel University Office of Institutional Advancement, Spring 2011.
38. Personal interview with George Buck, June 28, 2022.
39. "Q4 2009 NCO Group Earnings Conference Call," Fair Disclosure Wire, April 6, 2010, accessed via Gale OneFile: Business.
40. Cynthia Wilson, "Health Care Receivables Pose More Challenges Than Opportunities for Big Debt Collectors," InsideARM, March 7, 2011.
41. Blumenthal, "New CEO to Take Over."
42. Patrick Lunsford, "NCO Settles Debt Collection Action with 19 States," InsideARM, February 7, 2012.
43. *United States of America v. Expert Global Solutions, Inc.*, 3-13 CV2611-M (N. D. Texas).
44. DiStefano, "Despite Criticism, Debt Collector Keeps Expanding."
45. Federal Trade Commission, "The Structure and Practices of the Debt Buying Industry," January 2013, Table D2, https://www.ftc.gov/reports/structure-practices-debt-buying-industry.
46. Gideon Weissman et al., "Medical Debt Malpractice: Consumer Complaints About Medical Debt Collectors, and How the CFPB Can Help," US PIRG Education Fund and Frontier Group, 2017, 8.
47. "Expert Global Solutions Completes Sale of Certain Segments of Accounts Receivables Management Business to Platinum Equity," *Globe Newswire*, November 3, 2014.
48. "Tom Gores," *Forbes*, accessed July 15, 2022, https://www.forbes.com/profile/tom-gores/?sh=2804e2ab6b39.
49. After this sale, the medical debt collection was housed under the company Transworld Systems Inc. or TSI. "Expert Global Solutions to Sell Segments of

Accounts Receivables Management Business to Platinum Equity," Transworld Systems Inc., press release, July 14, 2014, https://www.platinumequity.com/news/expert-global-solutions-to-sell-segments-of-accounts.

50. "Platinum Equity Owned Transworld Systems Fined $2.5 Million for Illegal Student Debt Collection Lawsuits, Draws Thousands of Consumer Complaints," Private Equity Stakeholder Project, July 2019.

51. Gideon Weissman et al., "Medical Debt Malpractice," 16.

52. Consumer Complaint 5596439, May 24, 2022, CFPB Consumer Complaint Database.

53. Consumer Complaint 5387518, March 30, 2022, CFPB Consumer Complaint Database.

54. Consumer Complaint 3590300, April 2, 2020, CFPB Consumer Complaint Database.

55. Eileen Appelbaum and Rosemary Blatt, "Private Equity Buyouts in Healthcare: Who Wins, Who Loses," Institute for New Economic Thinking, Working Paper No. 118, March 15, 2020, 80.

56. Appelbaum and Blatt, "Private Equity Buyouts in Healthcare," 88.

57. Jerry Zremski, "Reed's Law Firm Operated Under His Name," Buffalo News, February 22, 2014.

58. Zremski, "Reed's Law Firm."

59. Brian Tumulty, "Reed Answers Ethics Questions," Democrat & Chronicle, February 24, 2014.

60. Lee Fang, "GOP Rep Tom Reed Founded Medical Debt Collection Firm That Harasses His Own Constituents," The Intercept, October 31, 2018.

61. Josh Brokaw, "4 Years After Closing Law Office, Tom Reed's Name Still on Credit Reports from Family's Medical Debt Collections Agency," TruthSayers, October 24, 2018; also see Federal Trade Commission, complaint filed June 30, 2015, from Hallstead, Pennsylvania, https://www.documentcloud.org/documents/5018919-Thomas-Reed-RR-Resource-Recovery-Complaints.html.

62. Fang, "GOP Rep Tom Reed."

63. Fang, "GOP Rep Tom Reed."

64. August Erbacher, "Congressman Tom Reed Resigns, Effective Immediately, Following Sexual Misconduct Accusation," WKBW, May 10, 2022.

65. Capio Company website, accessed November 17, 2022, https://www.capiofi.com/company.

66. "Jim Richards: A Builder of Business and a Rebuilder of the Collection Industry," Capital Club Radio, March 9, 2016.

67. M. P. Pell, "Patients in Arrears Face Collectors: Agencies Buy Up Delinquent Accounts," Atlanta Journal-Constitution, June 5, 2011.

68. Samantha Liss, "When a Nonprofit Health System Outsources Its ER, Debt Collectors Follow," St. Louis Post-Dispatch, April 17, 2016.

69. "Capio Co-Founder and Chairman Jim Richards Earns Integrity Award from the Receivables Management Association," Capio News, February 27, 2019.

70. "Jim Richards," Capital Group Radio, March 9, 2016.

71. "Jim Richards," Capital Group Radio.

72. "Frequently Asked Questions," Capio website, https://www.capiofi.com/faq.

73. "Frequently Asked Questions," Capio website.

74. Personal interview with Mark Detrick, October 21, 2022.

75. Personal interview with Mark Detrick, October 21, 2022.

76. "Frequently Asked Questions," Capio website.

CHAPTER 4

1. Ray Lefton, "What's It Worth? Cost Shifting, a Practice That Can Often Result in Significant Financial Burden on Self-Pay Patients, Is Leading to Greater Scrutiny of Hospital Charging Practices," *Healthcare Financial Management* 57, no. 12 (2003): 60.
2. Mark Oppenheimer, "Oppenheimer on the Advocate," *New Haven Review*, December 3, 2013.
3. Paul Bass, "Predator on the Hill," *The New Haven Advocate*, May 31, 2001.
4. Rollins, "Uncharitable Care."
5. Rollins, "Uncharitable Care," 13.
6. Ahu Yildirmaz and Mita Goldar, "Garnishment: The Untold Story," The ADP Research Institute, 2014, https://www.adp.com/tools-and-resources/adp-resea rch-institute/insights/~/media/ri/pdf/garnishment-whitepaper.ashx.
7. Rollins, "Uncharitable Care," 13.
8. Paul Kiel and Jeff Ernthausen, "Debt Collectors Have Made a Fortune This Year. Now They're Coming for More," ProPublica, October 5, 2020.
9. Grace Rollins, "Yale, Don't Lien on Me: The Attack on Homeownership by the Yale–New Haven Health System and Yale School of Medicine," Connecticut Center for a New Economy, September 2003, 3.
10. Rollins, "Uncharitable Care," 13.
11. Susan Kovac, "Judgment-Proof Debtors in Bankruptcy," *American Bankruptcy Law Journal* 65, no. 5 (Fall 1991): 681.
12. Personal interview with Grace Rollins, April 25, 2022.
13. Lucette Lagnado, "Jeanette White Is Long Dead But Her Hospital Bill Lives On," *Wall Street Journal*, March 13, 2003.
14. Lucette Lagnado, "Twenty Years—And He Isn't Paying Any More," *Wall Street Journal*, April 1, 2003.
15. Michigan Law Review Editorial Board, "The Unnecessary Doctrine of Necessaries," *Michigan Law Review* 82, no. 7 (1984): 1767.
16. States that have repealed the spousal "doctrine of necessaries" or equivalent obligations include Alabama, Alaska, Arkansas, Florida, Georgia, Idaho, Maryland, Michigan, Mississippi, Utah, Vermont, and Washington. "Doctrine of Necessaries," https://www.bills.com/learn/debt/doctrine-of-necessaries.
17. Melissa Jacoby and Elizabeth Warren, "Beyond Hospital Misbehavior: An Alternative Account of Medical-Related Financial Distress," *Northwestern University Law Review* 100, no. 2 (2006): 567.
18. Bearden v. Georgia, 461 US 660 (1983).
19. American Civil Liberties Union, *A Pound of Flesh: The Criminalization of Private Debt*, 6.
20. American Civil Liberties Union, *A Pound of Flesh: The Criminalization of Private Debt*, 2018, 14–15, https://www.aclu.org/sites/default/files/field_document/022 118-debtreport.pdf.
21. Lucette Lagnado, "Hospitals Try Extreme Measures to Collect Their Overdue Debts: Patients Who Skip Hearings," *Wall Street Journal*, October 30, 2003.
22. Lagnado, "Hospitals Try Extreme Measures."
23. Lucette Lagnado, "Hospital Found 'Not Charitable' Loses Its Status as Tax Exempt," *Wall Street Journal*, February 19, 2004.
24. Dan Diamond, "A Tarnished Hospital Tries to Win Back Trust," *Politico*, December 31, 2017.

25. Lucette Lagnado, "Call It Yale v. Yale: Law-School Clinic Is Taking Affiliated Hospital to Court over Debt Collection Tactics," *Wall Street Journal*, November 14, 2003.
26. Lagnado, "Call It Yale v. Yale."
27. Lagnado, "Call It Yale v. Yale."
28. Lagnado, "Twenty Years—And He Isn't Paying Any More."
29. Lagnado, "Twenty Years—And He Isn't Paying Any More."
30. Lagnado, "Call It Yale v. Yale."
31. Diamond, "A Tarnished Hospital."
32. Robert Seifert, "The Demand Side of Financial Exploitation: The Case of Medical Debt," *Housing Policy Debate* 15, no. 3 (2010): 785–803, 794.
33. Lagnado, "Call It Yale v. Yale."
34. Personal interview with James Greenwood, May 9, 2022.
35. Personal interview with James Greenwood, May 9, 2022.
36. Personal interview with James Greenwood, May 9, 2022.
37. Personal interview with James Greenwood, May 9, 2022.
38. James Greenwood, statement at hearing before the Subcommittee on Oversight and Investigations, in US House of Representatives Committee on Energy and Commerce, *A Review of Hospital Billing and Collections Practices* (Washington DC: US Government Printing Office, 2004).
39. Greenwood, in US House of Representatives Committee on Energy and Commerce, *A Review of Hospital Billing and Collections Practices*.
40. Greenwood, in US House of Representatives Committee on Energy and Commerce, *A Review of Hospital Billing and Collections Practices*, 106–8.
41. Trevor Fetter, statement, in US House of Representatives Committee on Energy and Commerce, *A Review of Hospital Billing and Collections Practices* (Washington, DC: US Government Printing Office, 2004), 104.
42. Henry Waxman, Representative from California, statement, in US House of Representatives, *A Review of Hospital Billing and Collections Practices* (Washington, DC: US Government Printing Office, 2004).
43. Josh Moon, "Who Is KB Forbes? The Answer Isn't Hard to Find or All That Unexpected," *Alabama Political Reporter*, July 16, 2020. For a more sympathetic portrait of Forbes, see Donald Bartlett and James Steele, *Critical Condition: How Health Care in America Became Big Business—and Bad Medicine* (New York: Crown, 2005), 16–24.
44. Tamar Lando, "Pocket Protector: KB Forbes Is Defending Uninsured Patients. Never Mind Why," *Mother Jones*, May/June 2005.
45. Lando, "Pocket Protector."
46. Ron Shinkman, "An Interview with K.B. Forbes, Advocate for the Uninsured," Fierce Healthcare, January 19, 2015.
47. Lando, "Pocket Protector"; also see US House of Representatives Committee on Energy and Commerce, *A Review of Hospital Billing and Collections Practices*, 5.
48. Lando, "Pocket Protector."
49. Allan Hubbard, "Press Briefing by Al Hubbard on the President's Health Care Initiatives for 2006," George W. Bush White House Archives, February 1, 2006, https://georgewbush-whitehouse.archives.gov/news/releases/2006/02/20060 201-1.html.
50. Karen Davis et al., "How High Is Too High? Implications of High-Deductible Health Plans," The Commonwealth Fund, April 1, 2005, 1.
51. Personal interview with Ruth Lande, August 22, 2022.

52. Richard Haugh and Dagmara Scalise, "A Surge in Bad Debt," *Hospitals & Health Networks,* December 2003, 14.
53. Michelle Doty et al., "Seeing Red: Americans Driven into Debt by Bills," The Commonwealth Fund, August 2005.
54. Alison Galbraith et al., "Nearly Half of Families in High-Deductible Health Plans Whose Members Have Chronic Conditions Face Substantial Financial Burden," *Health Affairs* 30, no. 2 (2011): 322–31.
55. Personal interview with Ruth Lande, August 22, 2022.
56. White House Council of Economic Advisers, "The Profitability of Health Insurance Companies," March 2018.
57. Greg Iacurci, "Here's Why Health Savings Accounts Contribute to Inequality," CNBC, April 14, 2022.

CHAPTER 5

1. Google Ngram, a searchable database of words or phrases in printed sources, can be used to demonstrate this disparity. The phrase "medical debt" appeared with the greatest frequency in printed sources published in 2008. But even in that year, "health spending" appeared more than seven times more often.
2. George Packer, *The Unwinding: An Inner History of America* (New York: Farrar, Straus & Giroux, 2013), 345.
3. Teresa Sullivan et al., *The Fragile Middle Class: Americans in Debt* (New Haven, CT: Yale University Press, 2000).
4. David Himmelstein et al., "Illness and Injury as Contributors to Bankruptcy," *Health Affairs* 24, S1 (2005): W-5-63–73.
5. David Himmelstein et al., "Medical Bankruptcy in the United States, 2007: Results of a National Study," *American Journal of Medicine* 122, no. 8 (August 2009): 741–46.
6. Himmelstein et al., "Medical Bankruptcy."
7. Carlos Dobkin et al., "Myth and Measurement: The Case of Medical Bankruptcies," *New England Journal of Medicine* 378, no. 12 (2018): 1076–78.
8. "Obama's Remarks at the White House Health Care Forum," *New York Times,* March 5, 2009, https://www.nytimes.com/2009/03/05/us/politics/05obama-text.html.
9. Elizabeth Warren, "Sick and Broke," *Washington Post,* February 9, 2005.
10. President Barack Obama, "Remarks by the President to a Joint Session of Congress on Health Care," Obama White House, September 9, 2009, https://obamawhitehouse.archives.gov/the-press-office/remarks-president-a-joint-session-congress-health-care.
11. Raymond Kluender et al., "Medical Debt in the US, 2009–2020," *Journal of the American Medical Association* 326, no. 3 (2021): 250–56.
12. Kluender et al., "Medical Debt."
13. These states include Alabama, Florida, Georgia, Kansas, Mississippi, North Carolina, South Carolina, South Dakota, Tennessee, Texas, Wisconsin, and Wyoming. See "Status of State Medicaid Expansion Decisions: Interactive Map," Kaiser Family Foundation, accessed November 21, 2022, https://www.kff.org/medicaid/issue-brief/status-of-state-medicaid-expansion-decisions-interactive-map.
14. Meghana Ammula and Robin Rudowitz, "Fate of Medicaid Expansion and Filling the Coverage Gap May Once Again Depend on the Outcome of State Elections," Kaiser Family Foundation, August 17, 2022.

15. US Census Bureau, "2018 SIPP Data," 2022, https://www.census.gov/programs-surveys/sipp/data/datasets/2018-data/2018.html
16. Kluender et al., "Medical Debt."
17. Alison Kodjak, "Widowed Early, a Cancer Doctor Writes About the Harm of Medical Debt," NPR, August 10, 2017.
18. Kodjak, "Widowed Early."
19. Kodjak, "Widowed Early."
20. Maria Pisu et al., "Costs of Cancer Along the Care Continuum: What We Can Expect Based on Recent Literature," *Cancer* 124, no. 21 (2018): 4181–91.
21. Charles Grassley, in US Senate Committee on Finance, *The Pulse of Charitable Care and Community Benefits at Nonprofit Hospitals* (Washington, DC: US Government Printing Office, 2006).
22. Dan Weissmann, "A Legendary Lawyer Sued Hospitals for Price-Gouging Their Patients. And Got His Butt Handed to Him," *An Arm and a Leg* podcast, Season 6, Episode 2, September 2, 2021, https://armandalegshow.com/episode/a-legendary-lawyer-sued-hospitals-for-price-gouging-their-patients-and-got-his-butt-handed-to-him/.
23. Nancy Kane and William Wubbenhorst, "Alternative Funding Policies for the Uninsured: Exploring the Value of Hospital Tax Exemption," *Milbank Quarterly* 78, no. 2 (2000): 185–212, 199.
24. Mark Taylor, "Full-Court Press," *Modern Healthcare* 34 (2004): 32–33. He was not alone in this assessment. In 2007, David R Williamson, Divisional Chief Financial Officer of the Health Management Associates, Inc., parent of the Yakima Regional Medical and Cardiac Center in Washington state, wrote that financial counselors would "have a face to face conversation" with uninsured patients "to ensure that they understand if they are going to utilize an HMA hospital they will be responsible for paying a portion of their bill. . . . This is an initiative that is coming from the very top of the organization and is something that the company is counting on to partially turn the tide of indigent patients entering into our system." See Eleanor Hamburger, Plaintiff's Motion for Partial Summary Judgment, *Angela Lopez v. Health Management Associates, Inc.*, in the Superior Court for Yakima County, December 30, 2014, No. 13-2-03580-3.
25. "Q3 2004 NCO Group Earnings Conference Call," Fair Disclosure Wire, November 2, 2004, accessed via Gale OneFile: Business.
26. Weissmann, "A Legendary Lawyer Sued Hospitals."
27. Internal Revenue Service, Section 501(r)(4), Financial Assistance Policy and Emergency Medical Care Policy.
28. Ge Bai and David Hyman, "Tax Exemptions for Nonprofit Hospitals: It's Time Taxpayers Get Their Money's Worth," *STATNews*, April 5, 2021, https://www.statnews.com/2021/04/05/tax-exemptions-nonprofit-hospitals-bad-deal-taxpayers.
29. Ge Bai et al., "Analysis Suggests Government and Nonprofit Hospitals' Charity Care Is Not Aligned with Their Favorable Tax Treatment," *Health Affairs* 40, no. 4 (2021), 629–36.
30. Thomas O'Toole et al., "Medical Debt and Aggressive Debt Restitution Practices," *Journal of General Internal Medicine* 19 (2004): 772–78.
31. Octavian Carare et al., "Exploring the Connection Between Financial Assistance for Medical Care and Medical Collections," Consumer Financial Protection Bureau, August 24, 2022, https://www.consumerfinance.gov/about-us/blog/exploring-connection-between-financial-assistance-for-medical-care-and-medical-collections.

32. Internal Revenue Service, Section 501(r)(6), Billings and Collections.
33. Internal Revenue Service, Section 501(r)(6).
34. Rau, "Patients Eligible for Charity Care."
35. Jessica Silver-Greenberg and Katie Thomas, "They Were Entitled to Free Care. Hospitals Hounded Them to Pay," *New York Times*, September 24, 2022.
36. Dan Weissmann, "Viral TikTok Video Serves Up Recipe to 'Crush' Medical Debt," *An Arm and a Leg* podcast, Season 4, Episode 16, February 15, 2021, https://arm andalegshow.com/episode/dollar-for.
37. Dollar For website, https://dollarfor.org.
38. Centura's financial assistance policy asks for "any crowd-funding websites, social media accounts, or bank sponsored charity/gift fund set up to solicit funds to pay for expenses." See "Financial Assistance Program, Patients," Centura Health, accessed December 23, 2022, https://centura.widen.net/s/6t7wwwsppl/financ ial-assistance-policy(.
39. Personal interview with Jared Walker, August 11, 2022.
40. Personal interview with Jared Walker, August 11, 2022. For more on Jared Walker, see Weissmann, "Viral TikTok Video."
41. Personal interviews with Kristi Cushman and Desember Terry, September 28, 2022.
42. Weissmann, "Viral TikTok Video."
43. Personal interview with Ruth Lande, August 22, 2022.
44. Personal interviews with Kristi Cushman and Desember Terry, September 28, 2022. Of note, in 2019, Oregon enacted a new law that requires hospitals to screen for presumptive eligibility before referring a bill to a debt collection agency or charging interest on the debt. See Jared Walker and Eli Rushbanks, "Pointless Debt: How Oregon Hospitals Skirt Financial Assistance Laws to Charge Patients—Without Increasing Revenue," Dollar For, February 2023.
45. Vince Galloro, "Making the Best of a Bad (Debt) Situation; Healthcare Organizations Shake Up Their Policies in Light of Increased Scrutiny of Charity Care," *Modern Healthcare*, February 28, 2005, 40.
46. Anna Wilde Mathews et al., "Hospitals Often Don't Help Needy Patients, Even Those Who Qualify," *Wall Street Journal*, November 17, 2022.
47. For instance, in order to investigate hospital lawsuits against patients in a single county in Mississippi, the Mississippi Center for Investigative Reporting spent weeks going through filing cabinets in the county courthouse examining tens of thousands of court records. See "How We Did It: The Painful Price for Healthcare," Mississippi Center for Investigative Reporting, August 6, 2021, https://www.mississippicir.org/news/how-we-did-it. For an explanation of the challenge for health services researchers, see Blake Shultz et al., "Hospital Debt Collection Practices Require Urgent Reform," *Health Affairs Forefront*, May 2, 2022.
48. Zack Cooper et al., "Hospital Lawsuits over Unpaid Bills Increased 37 Percent in Wisconsin from 2001 to 2018," *Health Affairs* 40, no. 12 (2021): 1830–35.
49. Will Bruhn et al., "Prevalence and Characteristics of Virginia Hospitals Suing Patients and Garnishing Wages for Unpaid Medical Bills," *Journal of the American Medical Association*, 322, no. 7 (August 2019): 691–92.
50. Victor Villagra et al., "When Hospitals and Doctors Sue Their Patients: The Medical Debt Crisis Through a New Lens," Health Disparities Institute Issue Brief, June 2019, 4.

51. Caitlin Owens, "America's Biggest Hospitals vs. Their Patients," Axios, June 14, 2021.
52. AFL-CIO et al., "Taking Neighbors to Court: Johns Hopkins Hospital Medical Debt Lawsuits," May 2019, https://www.nationalnursesunited.org/sites/default/files/nnu/documents/Johns-Hopkins-Medical-Debt-report.pdf.
53. Hilltop Institute, "Community Benefit State Law Profile: Maryland," August 2019, https://hilltopinstitute.org/wp-content/uploads/hcbp/hcbp_docs/HCBP_CBL_MD.pdf.
54. AFL-CIO et al., "Taking Neighbors to Court."
55. Personal interview with Lorig Charkoudian, September 6, 2022. Also see Harold Cohen, "Maryland's All-Payor Hospital Payment System," Health Services Cost Review Commission, n.d., https://hscrc.maryland.gov/documents/pdr/General Information/MarylandAll-PayorHospitalSystem.pdf.
56. Fred Schulte and James Drew, "In Their Debt," *Baltimore Sun*, December 21, 2008.
57. AFL-CIO et al., "Taking Neighbors to Court," 5.
58. AFL-CIO et al., "Taking Neighbors to Court."
59. Kelly Gooch, "Protest at Johns Hopkins Hospital Targets Lawsuits Against Low-Income Patients," *Becker's Hospital Review*, July 22, 2019.
60. Michelle Limpe, "Protesters Advocate for Legislation to Alleviate Burden of Medical Debt Lawsuits," *Johns Hopkins News-Letter*, April 10, 2021.
61. "Delegate Lorig Charkoudian: Healthcare," Everyday Canvassing, YouTube video, https://www.youtube.com/watch?v=bp5GU5g2nwQ.
62. Maryland State Bill HB 1420, "Hospitals: Financial Assistance Policies and Bill Collections," 2020.
63. Alia Paavola, "Maryland Changes Medical Debt Collection Rules for Hospitals," *Becker's Hospital Review*, January 4, 2022.
64. "Maryland Healthcare Collection Bill Becomes Law," Accountsrecovery.net, June 8, 2021.
65. Jay Hancock and Elizabeth Lucas, "'UVA Has Ruined Us': Health System Sues Thousands of Patients, Seizing Paychecks and Putting Liens on Homes," *Washington Post*, September 9, 2019.
66. "Grave of Virginia Child AIDS Victim Gets Headstone," *Washington Post*, June 10, 1985.
67. Jay Hancock et al., "UVA Health Revamps Aggressive Debt Collection Practices After Report," *Washington Post*, September 13, 2019.
68. Marty Makary, *The Price We Pay: What Broke American Healthcare and How to Fix It* (New York: Bloomsbury, 2019), 41.
69. Personal interview with Melissa Jacoby, September 6, 2022.
70. "Medical Debt Turning Into Credit Card Debt," *St. Louis Post-Dispatch*, June 11, 2008.
71. Melissa Jacoby and Elizabeth Warren, "Beyond Hospital Misbehavior: An Alternative Account of Medical-Related Financial Distress," *Northwestern University Law Review* 100, no. 2 (2006): 535–84, 537.
72. Jacoby and Warren, "Beyond Hospital Misbehavior," 539.
73. Jacoby and Warren, 541.
74. As of 2022, Medicare regulations require a "reasonable collection effort" for Medicare bad debt, which should include at least five mailers and three calls to patients to collect co-payments and co-insurance. If those efforts prove unsuccessful, the debt can be written off and partially reimbursed by Medicare.

Hospitals are not required to assign this debt to a collections agency or sell it, although they are required to use the same collection efforts in collecting from Medicare patients as from other patients. See Jeff Wolf and Mike Passanante, "Medicare Bad Debt 101," *The Hospital Finance Podcast*, May 25, 2022, https://www.besler.com/insights/medicare-bad-debt-101/.

75. Jacoby and Warren, "Beyond Hospital Misbehavior," 576.

76. Jacoby and Warren, "Beyond Hospital Misbehavior," 571. Also see *Heartland Health Systems v. Chamberlin,* 871 S. W. 2d 8 (Mo Ct. App. 1993).

77. Jacoby and Warren, "Beyond Hospital Misbehavior," 583.

78. John Colombo, in US House of Representatives Committee on Ways and Means. *The Tax-Exempt Hospital Sector*. Washington, DC: US Government Printing Office, 2005, 87.

79. Josh Kosman, *The Buyout of America: How Private Equity Is Killing Jobs and Destroying the American Economy* (New York: Portfolio, 2010).

80. Wendi Thomas, "This Doctors Group Is Owned by a Private Equity Firm and Repeatedly Sued the Poor Until We Called Them," ProPublica, November 27, 2019.

81. Margot Sanger-Katz et al., "Mystery Solved: Private-Equity Backed Firms Are Behind Ad Blitz on 'Surprise Billing,'" *New York Times*, September 30, 2021.

82. Robert Seifert and Mark Rukavina, "Bankruptcy Is the Tip of a Medical-Debt Iceberg," *Health Affairs* 25, no. 2 (2006): W89–92.

83. Interview with George Buck, June 28, 2022.

84. Peggy O'Farrell, "Seeking a Cure for Medical Debt," *Cincinnati Enquirer*, May 4, 2008.

85. Alex Kacik, "Hospitals' Uncompensated Care Continues to Rise," *Modern Healthcare*, November 21, 2019.

86. Robin Cohen et al., "Health Insurance Coverage: Early Release of Estimates from the National Health Interview Survey, 2017," National Center for Health Statistics, May 2018.

87. "Average Annual Deductible per Enrolled Employee in Employer-Based Insurance for Single and Family Coverage," Kaiser Family Foundation, 2021, https://www.kff.org/other/state-indicator/average-annual-deductible-per-enrolled-employee-in-employer-based-health-insurance-for-single-and-family-coverage/?currentTimeframe=0&sortModel=%7B%22colId%22:%22Location%22,%22sort%22:%22asc%22%7D.

88. M. P. Pell, "Patients in Arrears Face Collectors: Agencies Buy Up Delinquent Accounts," *Atlanta Journal-Constitution*, June 5, 2011.

89. Sarah Kliff, "With Medical Bills Skyrocketing, More Hospitals Are Suing for Payment," *New York Times*, November 8, 2019.

90. Personal interview with George Buck, June 28, 2022.

91. Melissa Jacoby, "The Debtor-Patient Revisited," *Saint Louis University Law Journal* 51, no. 2 (2007): 322–23.

92. Jacoby, "The Debtor-Patient Revisited."

93. For a history of budget cuts in New York City's municipal hospitals during the 1970s, for instance, see George Aumoithe, "Dismantling the Safety Net Hospital: The Construction of 'Underutilization' and Scarce Public Hospital Care," *Journal of Urban History*, November 10, 2021, https://doi.org/10.1177/00961442211056971.

94. For an in-depth journalistic exploration of the financial struggles of a small nonprofit hospital, see Brian Alexander, *The Hospital: Life, Death and Dollars in a Small American Town* (New York: St. Martin's, 2021).

95. Ge Bai, Farah Yehia, and Gerard Anderson, "Charity Care Provision by US Nonprofit Hospitals," *JAMA Internal Medicine* 180, no. 4 (2020): 606–7.

96. Michael Wilkes and David Schriger, "Why Won't UC Clinics Serve Patients with State-Funded Health Insurance?," *Los Angeles Times*, April 4, 2022.

CHAPTER 6

1. Strike Debt, "First Communiqué: Invisible Army." In *Tidal: Occupy Theory, Occupy Strategy, Year II*, September 2012, 2, https://ia801009.us.archive.org/16/items/tidal_3/tidal_3.pdf.

2. Andrew Ross and Astra Taylor, "Rolling Jubilee Is a Spark—Not the Solution," *The Nation*, August 27, 2012.

3. Personal interview with Astra Taylor, August 18, 2022.

4. Eli Cook, "Can David Graeber Become the Marx of the Debtor Class?," *Raritan Quarterly* 33, no. 2 (2006): 83–100.

5. Ross and Taylor, "Rolling Jubilee."

6. Astra Taylor, *Remake the World: Essays, Reflections, Rebellions* (Chicago: Haymarket Books, 2021), 26 .

7. Taylor, *Remake the World*, 26.

8. Taylor, *Remake the World*, 27.

9. Personal interview with Jerry Ashton, June 25, 2022.

10. "Every seventh year you shall grant a remission of debts. And this is the manner of the remission: Every creditor shall remit the claim that is held against a neighbor, not exacting it, because the LORD's remission has been proclaimed" (Deuteronomy 15:1–2). According to Leviticus, every 50 years, land was returned to its original owners, and Israelites who had been sold into bondage were set free (Leviticus 25:10). The Bible, New Revised Standard Version Updated Edition. Also see David Graeber, *Debt: The First 5,000 Years* (New York: Melville House, 2014), 403.

11. David Graeber, "Occupy and Anarchism's Gift of Democracy," *The Guardian*, November 15, 2011.

12. Graeber, *Debt: The First 5,000 Years*, 390.

13. Sparky Abraham and Eli Massey, "Medical Debt Special with Astra Taylor with Elizabeth Bruenig," *Current Affairs* podcast, 64 mins, January 26, 2021, https://podcasts.apple.com/au/podcast/medical-debt-special-with-astra-taylor-and/id1384567205?i=1000506611568.

14. Annie Nova, "She's Been Pushing for Student Loan Forgiveness for a Decade. Now It Could Happen," CNBC, May 15, 2022.

15. Personal interview with Jerry Ashton, June 25, 2022. Ashton and colleagues at RIP Medical Debt also began, when possible, to buy debt directly from hospitals rather than through debt buyers. But RIP Medical Debt forgives the debt of low-income patients (with incomes less than 400 percent of the federal poverty level or with debts that account for five percent or more of annual income), many of whom should, one could argue, should have been granted financial assistance by the hospital.

16. Robert Goff and Jerry Ashton, *The Patient, the Doctor, the Bill Collector: A Medical Debt Survival Guide* (Kauai, Hawaii: Hoku House, 2016).

17. *Last Week Tonight with John Oliver*, Season 3, Episode 14, "Debt Buyers," HBO, June 5, 2016, https://www.youtube.com/watch?v=hxUAntt1z2c.

18. *Last Week Tonight with John Oliver*.

19. *Last Week Tonight with John Oliver*.

20. Jerry Ashton et al., *End Medical Debt: Curing America's $1 Trillion Unpayable Healthcare Debt* (Kauai, HI: Hoku House, 2018).
21. *Last Week Tonight with John Oliver*.
22. Marshall Allen, *Never Pay the First Bill: And Other Ways to Fight the Health Care System and Win* (New York: Portfolio, 2021), 123.
23. John W. Kennedy, "US Navy Vet/Social Entrepreneur Jerry Ashton Says End Veteran Medical Debt," Let's Rethink This, March 7, 2022.
24. Consumer Financial Protection Bureau, "Medical Debt Burden in the United States," February 2022, 19–20, https://files.consumerfinance.gov/f/documents/cfpb_medical-debt-burden-in-the-united-states_report_2022-03.pdf.
25. Chris Arnold, "Senator 'Astounded' That Nonprofit Hospitals Sue Poorest Patients," NPR, July 22, 2015.
26. Wendi Thomas, "A Tennessee Hospital Sues Its Own Employees When They Can't Pay Their Medical Bills," NPR, June 28, 2019.
27. American Civil Liberties Union, *A Pound of Flesh: The Criminalization of Private Debt*, 2018, https://www.aclu.org/sites/default/files/field_document/022118-debtreport.pdf.
28. Margot Sanger-Katz and Sydney Ember, "Bernie Sanders Calls for Eliminating Americans' Medical Debt," *New York Times*, September 21, 2019.
29. Sanger-Katz and Ember, "Bernie Sanders Calls for Eliminating Americans' Medical Debt."
30. Sanger-Katz and Ember, "Bernie Sanders Calls for Eliminating Americans' Medical Debt."
31. Personal interview with James Zadoorian, July 14, 2022.
32. M. P. Pell, "Patients in Arrears Face Collectors: Agencies Buy Up Delinquent Accounts," *Atlanta Journal-Constitution*, June 5, 2011.
33. Michael Klozotsky, "How a (Non-Apple) U.S. Patent Might Just Change the World," *Forbes*, July 31, 2012.
34. Amy Martino, "Tricap Technology Group's CEO Refuses to Wait for Opportunity to Knock," *Sync*, August 12, 2016.
35. Personal interview with James Zadoorian, July 14, 2022.
36. James Zadoorian et al., "Patient-Centric Aid in a Consumer-Driven Marketplace," *Healthcare Financial Management*, December 1, 2018.
37. Zadoorian et al., "Patient-Centric Aid."
38. ARxChange website, https://arxchange.com (accessed July 13, 2022).
39. Melissa Jacoby and Mirya Holman, "Managing Medical Bills on the Brink of Bankruptcy," *Yale Journal of Health Policy, Law and Ethics* 10, no. 2 (2010): 239–97, 283.
40. Eileen Appelbaum and Rosemary Blatt, "Private Equity Buyouts in Healthcare: Who Wins, Who Loses," Institute for New Economic Thinking, Working Paper No. 118, March 15, 2020, 89–91, https://www.ineteconomics.org/uploads/papers/WP_118-Appelbaum-and-Batt-2-rb-Clean.pdf.
41. Appelbaum Rosemary Blatt, "Private Equity Buyouts in Healthcare, , 89–93.
42. Shefali Luthra, "Bank Loans Signed in the Hospital Leave Patients Vulnerable," *Los Angeles Times*, February 21, 2018.
43. Luthra, "Bank Loans Signed in the Hospital."
44. Farah Hashim et al., "Characteristics of US Hospitals Using Extraordinary Collections Actions Against Patients for Unpaid Medical Bills: A Cross-Sectional Study," *BMJ Open* 12 (2022): e060501.

45. Dave Goldiner, "State Suspends Medical, Student Debt Collection," *New York Daily News*, March 18, 2020.
46. Letitia James, "Attorney General James Renews Suspension of State Debt Collection for 10th Time as Coronavirus Continues to Impact New Yorkers' Wallets," press release, New York State Office of the Attorney General, February 1, 2021.
47. Brian Rosenthal, "One Hospital System Sued 2500 Patients After Pandemic Hit," *New York Times*, January 5, 2021.
48. Matt Mencarini, "Medical Debt Collection Continues Amid Pandemic," *Cincinnati Enquirer*, July 24, 2020, A4.
49. Matt Mencarini, "Medical Debt Collection Continues Amid Pandemic," *Cincinnati Enquirer*, July 24, 2020, A4.
50. Molly Castle Work, "They Could Have Qualified for Charity Care. But Mayo Clinic Sued Them," *Rochester Post-Bulletin*, November 22, 2022.
51. US Congress, Senate, "COVID-19 Medical Debt Collection Relief Act of 2021," S.355, 117th Congress, 1st sess., introduced in Congress February 22, 2021, https://www.govinfo.gov/app/details/BILLS-117s355is.
52. Cheryl Winkour Munk, "New Debt-Collection Rules: What They Mean for Consumers," *Wall Street Journal*, January 7, 2022.
53. Consumer Financial Protection Bureau, "Medical Debt Burden in the United States."
54. Anastassia Gliadkovskaya, "Consumer Financial Protection Bureau Examines Pitfalls in US Medical Billing," Fierce Healthcare, March 3, 2022.
55. Becky Yerak, "Medical Debt Collection, Reporting Under Scrutiny," *Chicago Tribune*, December 11, 2014.
56. Amy Traub, "Credit Reports and Employment: Findings from the 2012 National Survey on Credit Card Debt of Low- and Middle-Income Households," *Suffolk University Law Review* 46 (2013): 983–95, 983.
57. Kenneth Brevoort and Michelle Kambara, "Data Point: Medical Debt and Credit Scores," Consumer Financial Protection Bureau, May 2014, https://www.cons umerfinance.gov/data-research/research-reports/data-point-medical-debt-and-credit-scores.
58. Lisa Rowan, "70% of Medical Collection Debt Will Soon Be Removed from Credit Reports: Here's What You Need to Know," *Forbes*, April 5, 2022.
59. "Fact Sheet: The Biden Administration Announces New Actions to Lessen the Burden of Medical Debt and Increase Consumer Protection," The White House, April 11, 2022, https://www.whitehouse.gov/briefing-room/statements-releases/2022/04/11/fact-sheet-the-biden-administration-announces-new-actions-to-les sen-the-burden-of-medical-debt-and-increase-consumer-protection.
60. Kamala Harris, "Remarks by Vice President Harris Announcing Actions to Reduce the Burden of Medical Debt on American Families," The White House, April 11, 2022, https://www.whitehouse.gov/briefing-room/speeches-remarks/2022/04/11/remarks-by-vice-president-harris-announcing-actions-to-reduce-the-burden-of-medical-debt-on-american-families.

CONCLUSION

1. Michael Otremba, Gretchen Berland, and Joseph Amon, "Hospitals as Debtor Prisons," *Lancet Global Health* 3, no. 5 (2015): e253–54. Also see Robert Yates et al., "Hospital Detentions for Non-Payment of Fees: A Denial of Rights and Dignity," Chatham House Centre on Global Health Security, December 2017.

2. Marty Makary, *The Price We Pay: What Broke American Healthcare and How to Fix It* (New York: Bloomsbury, 2019), 48–49.

3. Dave Chokshi and Adam Beckman, "A New Category of 'Never Events'—Ending Harmful Hospital Policies," *JAMA Health Forum* 3, no. 10 (2022): e224703.

4. Victor Villagra et al., "When Hospitals and Doctors Sue Their Patients: The Medical Debt Crisis Through a New Lens," Health Disparities Institute Issue Brief, June 2019 6.

5. Avalere Health, "COVID-19's Impact on Acquisitions of Physician Practices and Physician Employment, 2019–2021," Physicians Advocacy Institute, April 2022, http://www.physiciansadvocacyinstitute.org/Portals/0/assets/docs/PAI-Resea rch/PAI%20Avalere%20Physician%20Employment%20Trends%20Study%202 019-21%20Final.pdf.

6. Ron Judd, "ER Doctor Who Criticized Bellingham Hospital's Coronavirus Protections Has Been Fired," *Seattle Times*, March 27, 2020.

7. Arthur Gale, "I Stuffed Their Mouths with Gold: How Hospitals Destroyed the Private Practice of Internal Medicine," *Missouri Medicine* 114, no. 1 (2017): 13–15. Also see Charles Webster, "Note on 'Stuffing their Mouths with Gold'," in *Aneurin Bevan on the National Health Service* (Oxford: Wellcome Unit for the History of Medicine, 1991), 219–21.

8. Richard Gunderman, "Medicine and the Pursuit of Wealth," *Hastings Center Report* 28, no. 1 (1998), 9–10.

9. Melissa Jacoby and Elizabeth Warren, "Beyond Hospital Misbehavior: An Alternative Account of Medical-Related Financial Distress," *Northwestern University Law Review* 100, no. 2 (2006): 535–84.

10. Christopher Robertson et al., "New State Consumer Protections Against Medical Debt," *Journal of the American Medical Association* 327, no. 2 (2022): 121–122.

11. Noam Levey, "Investigation: Many US Hospitals Sue Patients for Debts or Threaten Their Credit," NPR, December 21, 2022.

12. Thomas Rice et al., "Revisiting Out-of-Pocket Requirements: Trends in Spending, Financial Access Barriers, and Policy in Ten High-Income Countries," *BMC Health Services Research* 18, no. 18 (2018): 371.

13. Amitabh Chandra et al., "The Health Costs of Cost-Sharing," National Bureau of Economic Research, Working Paper 28439, February 2021.

14. Kenneth Arrow, "Uncertainty and the Welfare Economics of Medical Care," *American Economic Review* 53, no. 5 (1963), 941–947.

15. Mark Rukavina, statement before the Subcommittee on Oversight and Investigations, US House of Representatives Committee on Energy and Commerce, *A Review of Hospital Billing and Collections Practices* (Washington, DC: US Government Printing Office, 2004).

16. Antico's estimate, that all past-due medical debt could be purchased for $500 million, would represent less than one one-hundredth of 1 percent of federal spending in fiscal year 2022. See US Department of the Treasury, "Fiscal Data," n.d., https://fiscaldata.treasury.gov/americas-finance-guide/federal-spend ing/#federal-spending-overview.

17. Amanda Holpuch, "Medical Debt Is Being Erased in Ohio and Illinois. Is Your Town Next?," *New York Times*, December 29, 2022.

18. Astra Taylor, *Remake the World: Essays, Reflections, Rebellions* (Chicago: Haymarket Books, 2021).

19. William Beveridge, *Social Insurance and Allied Services. Inter-departmental Committee on Social Insurance and Allied Services* (London: His Majesty's Stationery Office, 1942), 158–59.
20. Paul Farmer, "Who Lives and Who Dies?," *London Review of Books*, February 5, 2015.
21. Ke Xu et al., "Protecting Households from Catastrophic Health Spending," *Health Affairs* 26, no. 4 (2007): 972.
22. Paul Farmer, "Health and Social Justice," lecture, Harvard University, Cambridge, MA, September 8, 2014.
23. Kelly Gooch, "Americans Struggle More with Medical Debt Than People in Other Countries, LA Times Reports," *Becker's Hospital Review*, September 13, 2019.
24. Margaret Atwood, *Payback: Debt and the Shadow Side of Wealth* (Toronto: House of Anansi Press, 2008), 52.
25. Sara Allin et al., "International Health Care System Profiles: Canada," The Commonwealth Fund, June 5, 2020.
26. Ross Tikkanen et al., "International Health Care System Profiles: Germany," The Commonwealth Fund, June 5, 2020.
27. Noam Levey, "Americans' Struggles with Medical Bills Are a Foreign Concept in Other Countries," *Los Angeles Times*, September 12, 2019.
28. "Medicare-for-All Prevents Medical Bankruptcies," Public Citizen, n.d., accessed January 15, 2023, https://www.citizen.org/article/medicare-for-all-prevents-medical-bankruptcies.
29. Linley Sanders, "Comparing American and British Attitudes on Health Care in 2022," YouGov, October 24, 2022.
30. Douglas Sherlock, "Indigent Care in Rational Markets," *Inquiry* 23 (Fall 1986): 261–67.
31. American Public Health Association, "Adopting a Single-Payer Health System," *Policy Statement Database*, Policy Number 20219, October 26, 2021.
32. John Nichols, "Obama's 'Eager to See' Better Approach on Health Reform," *The Nation,* January 28, 2010.
33. See, for instance, Paul Krugman, "Don't Make Health Care a Purity Test," *New York Times*, March 21, 2019.
34. Ronan Burtenshaw, "How the NHS Was Won," *Tribune Magazine*, May 7, 2019.
35. Sarah Kliff, "The Doctor's Strike That Nearly Killed Canada's Medicare-for-all Plan, Explained," *Vox*, March 29, 2019.
36. Nancy Ochieng et al., "Medicare-Covered Older Adults Are Satisfied with Their Coverage," Kaiser Family Foundation, May 17, 2021; K. Robin Yabroff et al., "Prevalence and Correlates of Medical Financial Hardship in the USA," *Journal of General Internal Medicine* 34, no. 8 (2019): 1494–1502.

AFTERWORD: MY DAY IN COURT

1. Jean-Paul Liranzo, Google review of Kent County Superior Court, Warwick, RI, 2021, accessed January 15, 2023, https://www.google.com/search?gs_ssp=eJwVx0EKgCAQAEC61ie8eE7NsvUJ_aIWCwksthXt99Hcpu36o9e8u5cgqcZLVWcI1m7O4Igazeq8qoNC3EEDuNnqacRFniGxwCsnfsWT70Dxov_EoqxUIp6C4gfUgB0U&q=kent+county+superior+court+warwick+ri&oq=kent+county+superiour+court+war&aqs=chrome.1.69i57j46i13i175i199i512.12956j0j7&sourceid=chrome&ie=UTF-8#lrd=0x89e44b72c5c1c2a7:0x30ccf9199784165c.
2. *Miriam Hospital v. Grajales*, 6SC-2017-00360, 2017, 6th Division District Court, Rhode Island.

3. *Newport Hospital v. Wicks*, 2SC-2017-00145, 2017, 2nd Division District Court, Rhode Island.

4. Personal interview with Mark Detrick, October 21, 2022.

5. *Miriam Hospital v. Tellier*, 3SC-2017-00447, 2017, 3rd Division District Court, Rhode Island.

6. *Rhode Island Hospital v. Johnson*, 6SC-2017-962, 2017, 6th Division District Court, Rhode Island.

7. Brian Jones, *Healing Rhode Island: The Story of Rhode Island Hospital, 1863–2013* (East Providence, RI: Signature Printing, 2013).

8. Emile Durkheim, *Elementary Forms of Religious Life*, trans. Karen Fields (Florence, MA: Free Press, 1995).

9. "And he entered the temple and began to drive out those who were selling and those who were buying in the temple, and he overturned the tables of the money changers and the seats of those who sold doves, and he would not allow anyone to carry anything through the temple. He was teaching and saying, 'Is it not written, "My house shall be called a house of prayer for all the nations"? But you have made it a den of robbers.'" The Bible, New Revised Standard Version Updated Edition (Mark 11: 15–17).

10. Paul Farmer, "We Know How to Confront the Coronavirus Pandemic—Expert Mercy," *Boston Globe*, March 19, 2020.

11. For more on this issue, see Devesh Kapur, "Philanthropy, Self-Interest, and Accountability: American Universities and Developing Countries," in *Giving Well: The Ethics of Philanthropy*, eds. Patricia Illingworth, Thomas Pogge, and Leif Weinar (Oxford: Oxford University Press, 2011), 285.

12. Sun Tzu, *The Art of War*, trans. Lionel Giles (New York: Dover, 2002).

13. Luke Messac, "Lifespan, Stop Suing My Patients," *UpriseRI*, September 19, 2019. For more on Lifespan finances and CEO compensation ($2,217,856 in reportable compensation from the organization in 2017, not including other compensation from the organization and related organizations), see the 2017 Form 990 for Lifespan Corporation, available on Guidestar.

14. Lifespan Corporation Services, "Lifespan Corporation and Affiliates Employee Social Media Policy," revised March 22, 2016.

15. Lifespan Corporation Services, "Lifespan Corporation and Affiliates Employee Social Media Policy."

16. ARS Collections website, accessed December 27, 2022, http://www.arscollection sri.com.

17. ARS Collections website.

18. Vince Galloro, "Making the Best of a Bad (Debt) Situation; Healthcare Organizations Shake Up Their Policies in Light of Increased Scrutiny of Charity Care," *Modern Healthcare*, February 28, 2005, 40.

19. "Medical Debt Policy Scorecard," Innovation for Justice, University of Arizona and University of Utah, accessed December 10, 2022, https://medicaldebtpoli cyscorecard.org.

BIBLIOGRAPHY

INTERVIEWS
Jerry Ashton, June 25, 2022.
George Buck, June 28, 2022.
CFPB Staff, December 12, 2022.
Lorig Charkoudian, September 6, 2022.
Kristi Cushman, September 28, 2022.
Mark Detrick, October 21, 2022
James Greenwood, May 9, 2022.
David Himmelstein, September 6, 2022.
Melissa Jacoby, September 6, 2022.
Ruth Lande, August 22, 2022.
Grace Rollins, April 25, 2022.
Astra Taylor, August 18, 2022.
Desember Terry, September 28, 2022.
Jared Walker, August 11, 2022.
James Zadoorian, July 14, 2022.

COMPANY WEBSITES AND EARNINGS CALLS
Account Recovery Services, https://www.arscollectionsri.com
ARS National Services, https://www.arsnational.com
ARxChange, https://arxchange.com
Capio, https://capio.com
Encore Capital Group, https://www.encorecapital.com
NCO Financial Systems, http://www.ncogroup.com
Transworld Systems, Inc., https://tsico.com

CONGRESSIONAL HEARINGS AND GOVERNMENT REPORTS
Anderson, Olin W. "National Consumer Survey of Medical Costs and Voluntary
    Health Insurance." In *Health Inquiry: Hearings Before the Committee on
    Interstate and Foreign Commerce, House of Representatives*. Washington, DC: US
    Government Printing Office, 1954, 2019–2131.
Beveridge, William. *Social Insurance and Allied Services. Inter-Departmental Committee
    on Social Insurance and Allied Services*. London: His Majesty's Stationery
    Office, 1942.
Brevoort, Kenneth, and Michelle Kambara. "Data Point: Medical Debt and Credit
    Scores." Consumer Financial Protection Bureau, May 2014. https://www.cons

umerfinance.gov/data-research/research-reports/data-point-medical-debt-
and-credit-scores

Carare, Octavian, Susan Singer, and Eric Wilson. "Exploring the Connection Between
Financial Assistance for Medical Care and Medical Collections." Consumer
Financial Protection Bureau blog, August 24, 2022. https://www.consumerfina
nce.gov/about-us/blog/exploring-connection-between-financial-assistance-for-
medical-care-and-medical-collections

"Chuck Piola," Catholic Speakers Organization Profiles, accessed January 14, 2023,
https://catholicspeakers.com/profiles/chuck-piola

Consumer Financial Protection Bureau. "Consumer Complaint Database." n.d.
https://www.consumerfinance.gov/data-research/consumer-complaints

Consumer Financial Protection Bureau. "Medical Debt Burden in the United States."
February 2022. https://files.consumerfinance.gov/f/documents/cfpb_medical-
debt-burden-in-the-united-states_report_2022-03.pdf

Consumer Financial Protection Bureau. "Study of Third-Party Debt Collection
Operations." July 2016. https://www.consumerfinance.gov/data-research/
research-reports/study-third-party-debt-collection-operations

Cooper, Cheryl. "The Debt Collection Market and Selected Policy Issues."
Congressional Research Service Report R46477, June 22, 2021. https://sgp.fas.
org/crs/misc/R46477.pdf

"Fact Sheet: The Biden Administration Announces New Actions to Lessen the Burden
of Medical Debt and Increase Consumer Protection." The White House, April
11, 2022. https://www.whitehouse.gov/briefing-room/statements-releases/
2022/04/11/fact-sheet-the-biden-administration-announces-new-actions-to-
lessen-the-burden-of-medical-debt-and-increase-consumer-protection

Federal Trade Commission. "The Structure and Practices of the Debt Buying
Industry." January 2013. https://www.ftc.gov/sites/default/files/documents/
reports/structure-and-practices-debt-buying-industry/debtbuyingreport.pdf

Frechtling, John, and Irving Schweiger. "1952 Survey of Consumer Finances, Part
III: Income, Selected Investments and Short-Term Debt of Consumers." *Federal
Reserve Bulletin* (September 1952): 974–1001. https://fraser.stlouisfed.org/
title/federal-reserve-bulletin-62/september-1952-21213

Furman, Jason, and Matt Fielder. "2014 Has Seen Largest Coverage Gains in Four
Decades, Putting the Uninsured Rate at or Near Historic Lows." Obama White
House Blog, December 18, 2014. https://obamawhitehouse.archives.gov/blog/
2014/12/18/2014-has-seen-largest-coverage-gains-four-decades-putting-
uninsured-rate-or-near-his

Harris, Kamala. "Remarks by Vice President Harris Announcing Actions to Reduce
the Burden of Medical Debt on American Families." The White House, April 11,
2022. https://www.whitehouse.gov/briefing-room/speeches-remarks/2022/
04/11/remarks-by-vice-president-harris-announcing-actions-to-reduce-the-bur
den-of-medical-debt-on-american-families

Henderson, Leon. *The Use of Small Loans for Medical Expenses*. Washington,
DC: Committee on the Costs of Medical Care, 1930.

Hubbard, Allan. "Press Briefing by Al Hubbard on the President's Health Care
Initiatives for 2006." George W. Bush White House Archives, February 1, 2006.
https://georgewbush-whitehouse.archives.gov/news/releases/2006/02/20060
201-1.html

Internal Revenue Service. "Rev. Rul. 56–185, 1956–1 C.B. 202." 1956. https://www.irs.
gov/pub/irs-tege/rr56-185.pdf

Internal Revenue Service. "Section 501(r)(4). Financial Assistance Policy and Emergency Medical Care Policy." n.d. https://www.irs.gov/charities-non-profits/financial-assistance-policy-and-emergency-medical-care-policy-section-501r4

Jackson, Andrew. "Third Annual Message, December 6, 1831." The American Presidency Project, n.d. https://www.presidency.ucsb.edu/documents/third-annual-message-3

James, Letitia. "Attorney General James Renews Suspension of State Debt Collection for 10th Time as Coronavirus Continues to Impact New Yorkers' Wallets." Press release, New York State Office of the Attorney General, February 1, 2021.

Johnson, Lyndon B. "Remarks with President Truman at the Signing in Independence of the Medicare Bill, July 30, 1965." The American Presidency Project, n.d. https://www.presidency.ucsb.edu/documents/remarks-with-president-truman-the-signing-independence-the-medicare-bill

Lifespan Corporation. "Form 990: Return of Organization Exempt from Income Tax." 2017.

Obama, Barack. "Remarks at the White House Health Care Forum, March 5, 2009." Obama White House, March 30, 2009. https://obamawhitehouse.archives.gov/blog/2009/03/30/white-house-forum-health-reform-report

Obama, Barack. "Remarks by the President to a Joint Session of Congress on Health Care." Obama White House, September 9, 2009. https://obamawhitehouse.archives.gov/the-press-office/remarks-president-a-joint-session-congress-health-care

Reagan, Ronald. "The President's News Conference, November 10, 1981." Ronald Reagan Presidential Library & Museum, n.d. https://www.reaganlibrary.gov/archives/speech/presidents-news-conference

US Census Bureau. "2018 SIPP Data." 2022. https://www.census.gov/programs-surveys/sipp/data/datasets/2018-data/2018.html

US Census Bureau. "2018 Survey of Income and Program Participation Datasets." 2022. https://www.census.gov/programs-surveys/sipp/data/datasets.2018.html#list-tab-OVR8G0IJZM8P0I5TJK

U.S. Congress, Senate, "COVID-19 Medical Debt Collection Relief Act of 2021." S.355, 117th Congress, 1st sess., introduced in Congress February 22, 2021. https://www.govinfo.gov/app/details/BILLS-117s355is

US Department of Health, Education, and Welfare. *Medical Care in Transition, Volume 2*. Washington, DC: US Government Printing Office, 1964.

US Department of the Treasury. "Fiscal Data." n.d. https://fiscaldata.treasury.gov/americas-finance-guide/federal-spending/#federal-spending-overview

US House of Representatives Committee on Energy and Commerce. *A Review of Hospital Billing and Collections Practices*. Washington, DC: US Government Printing Office, 2004. https://www.govinfo.gov/content/pkg/CHRG-108hhrg95446/html/CHRG-108hhrg95446.htm

US House of Representatives Committee on Ways and Means. *The Tax-Exempt Hospital Sector*. Washington, DC: US Government Printing Office, 2005. https://www.govinfo.gov/content/pkg/CHRG-109hhrg26414/html/CHRG-109hhrg26414.htm

US Senate Committee on Finance. *The Pulse of Charitable Care and Community Benefits at Nonprofit Hospitals*. Washington, DC: US Government Printing Office, 2006.

US Senate Subcommittee on Financial Institutions and Consumer Protection of the Committee on Banking, Housing and Urban Affairs. *Shining a Light on the*

Consumer Debt Industry. S. Hrg. 113-75, July 17, 2013. https://www.govinfo.
    gov/app/details/CHRG-113shrg82718
White House Council of Economic Advisers. "The Profitability of Health Insurance
    Companies." March 2018.

NONGOVERNMENTAL REPORTS
"1 in 10 Adults Owe Medical Debt, with Millions Owing More Than $10,000."
    Kaiser Family Foundation, March 10, 2022. https://www.kff.org/hea
    lth-costs/press-release/1-in-10-adults-owe-medical-debt-with-milli
    ons-owing-more-than-10000
"A Brief History of Debt Collection and Its Regulation in the United States." National
    Consumer Law Center Digital Library, 2022. Accessed January 12, 2023, from
    https://library.nclc.org/book/fair-debt-collection/12-brief-history-debt-collect
    ion-and-its-regulation-united-states
ACA International. "Diversity in the Collections Industry: Examining the
    Demographics of Collection Agents." 2022. https://www.acainternational.org/
    wp-content/uploads/2022/08/Diversity-in-the-Collections-Industry-2022-
    FinalACA.pdf
The Access Project. "The Consequences of Medical Debt: Evidence from Three
    Communities." February 2003. https://www.healthcareconsumers.org/files/
    med_consequences.pdf
AFL-CIO, National Nurses United, and Coalition for a Humane Hopkins. "Taking
    Neighbors to Court: Johns Hopkins Hospital Medical Debt Lawsuits." May
    2019. https://www.nationalnursesunited.org/sites/default/files/nnu/docume
    nts/Johns-Hopkins-Medical-Debt-report.pdf
Allin, Sara, Greg Marchildon, and Allie Peckham. "International Health Care System
    Profiles: Canada." Commonwealth Fund, June 5, 2020. https://www.commo
    nwealthfund.org/international-health-policy-center/countries/canada
American Civil Liberties Union. *A Pound of Flesh: The Criminalization of Private Debt*.
    2018. https://www.aclu.org/sites/default/files/field_document/022118-deb
    treport.pdf
American Hospital Association. "Fast Facts on US Hospitals, 2022." 2022. https://
    www.aha.org/system/files/media/file/2022/01/fast-facts-on-US-hospitals-
    2022.pdf
American Public Health Association, "Adopting a Single-Payer Health System," Policy
    Statement Database, Policy Number 20219, October 26, 2021, https://www.
    apha.org/Policies-and-Advocacy/Public-Health-Policy-Statements/Policy-
    Database/2022/01/07/Adopting-a-Single-Payer-Health-System
"Americans' Views of Healthcare Costs, Coverage and Policy." Westhealth Institute,
    2018. https://www.norc.org/PDFs/WHI%20Healthcare%20Costs%20Cover
    age%20and%20Policy/WHI%20Healthcare%20Costs%20Coverage%20and%20
    Policy%20Issue%20Brief.pdf
Ammula, Meghana, and Robin Rudowitz. "Fate of Medicaid Expansion and Filling the
    Coverage Gap May Once Again Depend on the Outcome of State Elections."
    Kaiser Family Foundation, August 17, 2022. https://www.kff.org/policy-watch/
    fate-of-medicaid-expansion-and-filling-the-coverage-gap-may-once-again-dep
    end-on-the-outcome-of-state-elections
Avalere Health. "COVID-19's Impact on Acquisitions of Physician Practices and
    Physician Employment, 2019–2021." Physicians Advocacy Institute, April
    2022. http://www.physiciansadvocacyinstitute.org/Portals/0/assets/docs/

PAI-Research/PAI%20Avalere%20Physician%20Employment%20Trends%20St
udy%202019-21%20Final.pdf

"Average Annual Deductible per Enrolled Employee in Employer-Based Insurance for
Single and Family Coverage." Kaiser Family Foundation, 2021. https://www.
kff.org/other/state-indicator/average-annual-deductible-per-enrolled-emplo
yee-in-employer-based-health-insurance-for-single-and-family-coverage/
?currentTimeframe=0&sortModel=%7B%22colId%22:%22Location%22,%22s
ort%22:%22asc%22%7D

"Bad Debt Exceeds $10M at a Third of Organizations, But Lack of Confidence Exists
in How Much Is Recoverable." Sage Growth Partners, June 19, 2018. https://
sage-growth.com/index.php/news/press-release-bad-debt-exceeds-10m-third-
organizations-lack-confidence-exists-much-recoverable

Cohen, Robin, Emily Zammitti, and Michael Martinez. "Health Insurance
Coverage: Early Release of Estimates from the National Health Interview
Survey, January—March 2017." National Center for Health Statistics, May
2018. https://www.cdc.gov/nchs/data/nhis/earlyrelease/insur201708.pdf

Davis, Karen, Michelle Doty, and Alice Ho. "How High Is Too High? Implications
of High-Deductible Health Plans." The Commonwealth Fund, April 1, 2005.
https://www.commonwealthfund.org/publications/fund-reports/2005/apr/
how-high-too-high-implications-high-deductible-health-plans

"Debt Collection Agencies in the US, Number of Businesses 2005–2008." IBIS World,
June 28, 2022. https://www.ibisworld.com/industry-statistics/number-of-bus
inesses/debt-collection-agencies-united-states

"Disproportionate Share Hospital Payments." Medicaid and CHIP Payment and
Access Commission, n.d. https://www.macpac.gov/subtopic/disproportionate-
share-hospital-payments

Doty, Michelle, Jennifer Edwards, and Alyssa Holmgren. "Seeing Red: Americans
Driven into Debt by Medical Bills." The Commonwealth Fund, August 2005.
https://www.commonwealthfund.org/sites/default/files/documents/___
media_files_publications_issue_brief_2005_aug_seeing_red__americans_
driven_into_debt_by_medical_bills_837_doty_seeing_red_medical_d
ebt_pdf.pdf

Duchon, Lisa, Cathy Schoen, and Michelle Doty. "How Instability in Health Insurance
Puts U.S. Workers at Risk." The Commonwealth Fund, December 2001. https://
www.commonwealthfund.org/publications/fund-reports/2001/dec/security-
matters-how-instability-health-insurance-puts-us

Dunker, Amanda, and Elisabeth Ryden Benjamin. "Discharged into Debt: A Pandemic
Update." Consumer Service Society, Policy Brief, January 2021. https://www.
cssny.org/publications/entry/discharged-into-debt-a-pandemic-update

Federal Trade Commission. "Leading Debt Collector Agrees to Pay Record $2.8 Million
to Settle FTC Charges." Press release, March 16, 2011. https://www.ftc.gov/
news-events/news/press-releases/2011/03/leading-debt-collector-agrees-pay-
record-28-million-settle-ftc-charges

Grover, Michael. "What a $400 Emergency Expense Tells Us About the Economy."
Federal Reserve Bank of Minneapolis, June 11, 2021. https://www.minneap
olisfed.org/article/2021/what-a-400-dollar-emergency-expense-tells-us-about-
the-economy

Hilltop Institute. "Community Benefit State Law Profile: Maryland." August 2019.
https://hilltopinstitute.org/wp-content/uploads/hcbp/hcbp_docs/HCBP_CBL
_MD.pdf

"Hospital by Ownership Type: 2020." Kaiser Family Foundation, n.d. https://
    www.kff.org/other/state-indicator/hospitals-by-ownership/?currentTi
    meframe=0&sortModel=%7B%22colId%22:%22Location%22,%22s
    ort%22:%22asc%22%7D
"The Impact of Third-Party Debt Collection on the National and State Economies."
    Ernst & Young, January 2012. https://www.creditandcollectionnews.com/uplo
    ads/The%20Impact%20of%203rd%20Party%20Debt%20Collection%20on%20
    the%20National%20and%20State%20Economies.pdf
Kirzinger, Ashley, Cailey Muñana, Brian Wu, and Mollyann Brodie. "Data
    Note: Americans' Challenges with Health Care Costs." Kaiser Family
    Foundation, June 11, 2019. https://www.kff.org/health-costs/issue-brief/data-
    note-americans-challenges-health-care-costs/view/footnotes
Lifespan Corporation Services. "Lifespan Corporation and Affiliates Employee Social
    Media Policy," revised March 22, 2016.
"Medicare-for-All Prevents Medical Bankruptcies." Public Citizen, n.d. Accessed
    January 15, 2023. https://www.citizen.org/article/medicare-for-all-prevents-
    medical-bankruptcies
Mississippi Center for Investigative Reporting. "How We Did It: The Painful Price
    for Healthcare." August 6, 2021. https://www.mississippicir.org/news/
    how-we-did-it
Ochieng, Nancy, Jeannie Fulgeston Biniek, Karyn Schwartz, and Tricia Neuman.
    "Medicare-Covered Older Adults Are Satisfied with Their Coverage." Kaiser
    Family Foundation, May 17, 2021. https://www.kff.org/report-section/medic
    are-covered-older-adults-are-satisfied-with-their-coverage-have-similar-access-
    to-care-as-privately-insured-adults-ages-50-to-64-issue-brief
Perry, Andre, Carl Romer, and Nana Adjeiwaa-Manu. "The Racial Implications of
    Medical Debt: How Moving Toward Universal Health Care and Other Reforms
    Can Address Them." Brookings Institute, October 5, 2021.
"Platinum Equity Owned Transworld Systems Fined $2.5 Million for Illegal Student
    Debt Collection Lawsuits, Draws Thousands of Consumer Complaints." Private
    Equity Stakeholder Project, July 2019.
Rau, Jordan. "Patients Eligible for Charity Care Instead Get Big Bills." *Kaiser Health
    News*, October 14, 2019.
Reid, David. "The Debt Buying Industry." Receivables Management Association
    International White Paper, 2016. https://rmaintl.org/wp-content/uploads/
    2019/01/White-Paper-The-Debt-Buying-Industry_Executive_Summary.pdf
Rollins, Grace. "Uncharitable Care: Yale–New Haven Hospital's Charity Care and
    Collections Practices." Connecticut Center for a New Economy, January 2003.
Rollins, Grace. "Yale, Don't Lien on Me: The Attack on Homeownership by the Yale–
    New Haven Health System and Yale School of Medicine." Connecticut Center
    for a New Economy, September 2003.
"Social Welfare Under Reagan." CQ Researcher, March 9, 1984. https://library.cqpr
    ess.com/cqresearcher/document.php?id=cqresrre1984030900
"Status of State Medicaid Expansion Decisions: Interactive Map." Kaiser Family
    Foundation. Accessed November 21, 2022. https://www.kff.org/medicaid/
    issue-brief/status-of-state-medicaid-expansion-decisions-interactive-map
Strike Debt. "First Communiqué: Invisible Army." In *Tidal: Occupy Theory, Occupy
    Strategy, Year II.* September 2012. https://ia801009.us.archive.org/16/items/
    tidal_3/tidal_3.pdf

Strike Debt and Occupy Wall Street. "The Debt Resistors' Operations Manual."
September 2012. https://strikedebt.org/The-Debt-Resistors-Operations-Man
ual.pdf

Tikkanen, Ross, Robin Osborn, Elias Mossialos, Ana Djordjevic, and George Wharton.
"International Health Care System Profiles: Germany." The Commonwealth
Fund, June 5, 2020.

*Transactions of the Medical and Chirurgical Faculty of the State of Maryland, 91st
Annual Session, Held at Baltimore, Md. April 1889.* Baltimore: Press of Isaac
Friedenwald, 1889.

Walker, Jared, and Eli Rushbanks. "Pointless Debt: How Oregon Hospitals Skirt
Financial Assistance Laws to Charge Patients—Without Increasing Revenue."
Dollar For, February 2023.

Weissman, Gideon, Ed Mierzwinski, and Mike Litt. "Medical Debt
Malpractice: Consumer Complaints About Medical Debt Collectors, and How
the CFPB Can Help." US PIRG Education Fund and Frontier Group, 2017.

Yates, Robert, Tom Brookes, and Eloise Whitaker. "Hospital Detentions for Non-
Payment of Fees: A Denial of Rights and Dignity." Chatham House Centre on
Global Health Security, December 2017. https://www.chathamhouse.org/2017/
12/hospital-detentions-non-payment-fees

Yildermaz, Ahu, and Mita Goldar. "Garnishment: The Untold Story." ADP Research
Institute, 2014. https://www.adp.com/tools-and-resources/adp-research-instit
ute/insights/~/media/ri/pdf/garnishment-whitepaper.ashx

**PUBLISHED SOURCES (JOURNALS, BOOKS, PERIODICALS, AND ONLINE
PUBLICATIONS)**

Abraham, Sparky, and Eli Massey. "Medical Debt Special with Astra Taylor with
Elizabeth Bruenig." *Current Affairs* podcast, 64 mins, January 26, 2021.
https://podcasts.apple.com/au/podcast/medical-debt-special-with-astra-tay
lor-and/id1384567205?i=1000506611568

Acosta, Katherine. "Surviving the American Health Care System: Experiences and
Strategies of Uninsured Women." PhD diss., University of Nebraska, 2003.

Adams, Alyce, Raymond Kluender, Neale Mahoney, Jinglin Wang, Francis Wong,
and Wesley Yin. "The Impact of Financial Assistance Programs on Health Care
Utilization." National Bureau of Economic Research, Working Paper 29227,
August 31, 2021. https://www.hbs.edu/ris/PublicationFiles/22-045_16db6f8b-
1540-440c-bd62-588714a7e5b0.pdf

Ahles, Andrea. "Fort Washington, PA, Collection Agency Finds Profit in Others'
Debt." *Philadelphia Inquirer*, December 21, 1998.

Alexander, Brian. *The Hospital: Life, Death and Dollars in a Small American Town.*
New York: St. Martin's, 2021.

Allen, Marshall. *Never Pay the First Bill: And Other Ways to Fight the Health Care System
and Win.* New York: Portfolio, 2021.

Allison, Wes. "Working Cure." *Richmond Times-Dispatch*, March 20, 1995.

"Allowing Low-Income Hospital Patients to Work off Their Hospital Bills." *Healthcare
PR and Marketing News* 7, no. 5 (March 1998).

Anderson, Gerard. "From 'Soak the Rich' to 'Soak the Poor': Recent Trends in Hospital
Pricing." *Health Affairs* 26, no. 3 (2007): 780–89.

Anderson, Rozanne. "Powering up the Rev Cycle—Hot Topics for Healthcare
Providers." InsideARM, November 22, 2017.

Appelbaum, Eileen, and Rosemary Blatt. "Private Equity Buyouts in Healthcare: Who Wins, Who Loses." Institute for New Economic Thinking, Working Paper No. 118, March 15, 2020. https://www.ineteconomics.org/uploads/papers/WP_118-Appelbaum-and-Batt-2-rb-Clean.pdf

Arnold, Chris. "Senator 'Astounded' That Nonprofit Hospitals Sue Poorest Patients." NPR, July 22, 2015.

Arrow, Kenneth. "Uncertainty and the Welfare Economics of Medical Care." *American Economic Review* 53, no. 5 (1963): 941–73.

Ashton, Jerry, Robert Goff, and Craig Antico. *End Medical Debt: Curing America's $1 Trillion Unpayable Healthcare Debt.* Kauai, HI: Hoku House, 2018.

Atwood, Margaret. *Payback: Debt and the Shadow Side of Wealth.* Toronto: House of Anansi Press, 2008.

Aumoithe, George. "Dismantling the Safety Net Hospital: The Construction of 'Underutilization' and Scarce Public Hospital Care." *Journal of Urban History* (November 10, 2021). https://doi.org/10.1177/00961442211056971

Bai, Ge, and David Hyman, "Tax Exemptions for Nonprofit Hospitals: It's Time Taxpayers Get Their Money's Worth." *STATNews*, April 5, 2021. https://www.statnews.com/2021/04/05/tax-exemptions-nonprofit-hospitals-bad-deal-taxpayers

Ge Bai, Farah Yehia, and Gerard Anderson, "Charity Care Provision by US Nonprofit Hospitals," *JAMA Internal Medicine* 180, no. 4 (2020): 606-607.

Bai, Ge, Hossein Zare, Matthew Eisenberg, Daniel Polsky, and Gerard F. Anderson. "Analysis Suggests Government and Nonprofit Hospitals' Charity Care Is Not Aligned with Their Favorable Tax Treatment." *Health Affairs* 40, no. 4 (2021): 629–36.

Bannow, Tara. "Few Hospitals Aggressively Sue Patients to Pay Bills." *Modern Healthcare* (October 5, 2019).

Bartlett, Donald, and James Steele. *Critical Condition: How Health Care in America Became Big Business—and Bad Medicine.* New York: Crown, 2005.

Bass, Paul. "Heartless Hospital." *New Haven Advocate*, April 17, 2003.

Bass, Paul. "Predator on the Hill." *New Haven Advocate*, May 31, 2001.

Blumenthal, Jeff. "New CEO to Take over at Debt Collector NCO." *Philadelphia Business Journal*, March 21, 2011.

Boyd, Janice. "The Debt Buying Market Comes of Age." *Collector* 86, no. 12 (2021): 40–41.

Bradbury, Ray. *Fahrenheit 451.* New York: Ballantine, 1953.

Brokaw, Josh. "4 Years After Closing Law Office, Tom Reed's Name Still on Credit Reports from Family's Medical Debt Collections Agency." *TruthSayers*, October 24, 2018.

Bromberg, Robert. "The Charitable Hospital." *Catholic University Law Review* 20, no. 2 (1970): 237–58.

Bromberg, Robert. "Financing Health Care and the Effect of the Tax Law." *Law and Contemporary Problems* 39, no. 4 (1975): 156–82.

Bruhn, Will, Lainie Rutkow, Peiqi Wang, Stephen E. Tinker, Christine Fahim, Heidi N. Overton, and Martin A. Makary. "Prevalence and Characteristics of Virginia Hospitals Suing Patients and Garnishing Wages for Unpaid Medical Bills." *Journal of the American Medical Association* 322, no. 7 (2019): 691–92.

Burtenshaw, Ronan. "How the NHS Was Won." *Tribune Magazine*, May 7, 2019.

Callicoat, Jason, and David Rumbach. "Medical Debt Problem Requires Creative Thinking." *South Bend Tribune*, July 2, 2001.

Castle Work, Molly. "They Could Have Qualified for Charity Care. But Mayo Clinic Sued Them." *Rochester Post-Bulletin*, November 22, 2022.

Caswell, Kyle, and John Goddeeris. "Does Medicare Reduce Medical Debt?" *American Journal of Health Economics* 6, no. 1 (Winter 2020). doi:10.1086/706623

Cathell, Aniel Webster. *The Physician Himself from Graduation to Old Age.* Philadelphia: Davis, 1925.

Chandra, Amitabh, Evan Flack, and Ziad Obermeyer. "The Health Costs of Cost-Sharing." National Bureau of Economic Research, Working Paper 28439, February 2021. doi:10.3386/w28439

Chokshi, Dave, and Adam Beckman. "A New Category of 'Never Events'—Ending Harmful Hospital Policies." *JAMA Health Forum* 3, no. 10 (2022): e224703.

Clark, David. "Profits, Publicity Fuel Trend Toward Marketing of Health-Care Services." *Christian Science Monitor*, December 5, 1984

Cohen, Harold. "Maryland's All-Payor Hospital Payment System." Health Services Cost Review Commission, n.d. https://hscrc.maryland.gov/documents/pdr/GeneralInformation/MarylandAll-PayorHospitalSystem.pdf

Cohodes, Donald. "America: The Home of the Free, the Land of the Uninsured." *Inquiry* 23 (1986): 227–35.

Coleman, Peter. *Debtors and Creditors in America: Insolvency, Imprisonment for Debt, and Bankruptcy, 1607–1900.* Fairless Hills, PA: Beard Books, 1999.

Cook, Eli. "Can David Graeber Become the Marx of the Debtor Class?" *Raritan Quarterly* 33, no. 2 (2006): 83–100.

Cooper, Zack, James Han, and Neale Mahoney. "Hospital Lawsuits over Unpaid Bills Increased 37 Percent in Wisconsin from 2001 to 2018." *Health Affairs* 40, no. 12 (2021): 1830–35.

Crenshaw, Albert. "Bill Collectors' Abusive Tactics Under Scrutiny." *Washington Post*, September 13, 1992.

Crompton, Kim. "Spokane Hospitals Soft-Pedal Debt Collections." *Spokane Journal of Business* 7, no. 19 (October 1992): B3.

Cutler, David. "Cost Shifting or Cost Cutting? The Incidence of Reductions in Medicare Payments." In *Tax Policy and the Economy*, vol. 12, edited by James M. Poterba, 1–28. Cambridge, MA: MIT Press, 1998. http://www.nber.org/chapters/c10911

Cutler, David. "Equality Efficiency, and Market Fundamentals: The Dynamics of International Medical Reform." *Journal of Economic Literature* 40, no. 3 (2002): 881–906.

Cutler, David, Mark McClellan, and Joseph Newhouse. "How Does Managed Care Do It?" *Rand Journal of Economics* 31, no. 3 (2000): 526–48.

Darling, Helen. "The Role of the Federal Government in Assuring Access to Health Care." *Inquiry* 23, no. 3 (1986): 286–96.

"Delegate Lorig Charkoudian: Healthcare." Everyday Canvassing, YouTube video, https://www.youtube.com/watch?v=bp5GU5g2nwQ

Devitt, Caitlin. "A Debt Rx for Healthcare: Hospitals Are Dealing with More and More Bad Debt, Trying to Figure Out Whether and When They Should Sell and What Role Collection Should Pay." *Collections & Credit Risk* 11, no. 10 (2006): 34.

Devitt, Caitlin. "Medical Debt Heavy Hitters." *Collections & Credit Risk* 12, no. 5 (2007): 48–55.

Devitt, Caitlin. "Taking the Pulse on Healthcare Collections: How Will Healthcare Collections Change as Reform Plans Sweep the Country?" *Collections & Credit Risk* 12, no. 9 (2007): 18.Diamond, Dan. "A Tarnished Hospital Tries to Win Back Trust." *Politico*, December 31, 2017.

Dickens, Charles. *The Pickwick Papers*. Knoxville, TN: Wordsworth Classics, 1993 (1837).

DiStefano, Joseph. "Despite Criticism, Debt Collector Keeps Expanding." *Philadelphia Inquirer*, July 21, 2013.

Dobkin, Carlos, Amy Finkelstein, Raymend Kluender, and Matthew J. Notowidigdo. "Myth and Measurement: The Case of Medical Bankruptcies." *New England Journal of Medicine* 378, no. 12 (2018): 1076–78.

Dunbar, Paul Laurence. "The Debt." In *The Collected Poetry of Paul Laurence Dunbar*, edited by Joanne Braxton, 213. Charlottesville, University of Virginia Press, 1993.

Duncan, R. Paul, and Kerry Kilpatrick. "Unresolved Hospital Charges in Florida." *Health Affairs* 6, no. 1 (1987): 159–60.

Durkheim, Emile. *Elementary Forms of Religious Life*, trans. Karen Fields. Florence, MA: Free Press, 1995.

Erbacher, August. "Congressman Tom Reed Resigns, Effective Immediately, Following Sexual Misconduct Accusation." WKBW, May 10, 2022.

Ewing, Crystal. "Hospitals Seek Out New Ways to Reduce Bad Debt, Focus on Self-Pay Patients." *Becker's Hospital Review*, November 14, 2017.

"Expert Global Solutions Completes Sale of Certain Segments of Accounts Receivables Management Business to Platinum Equity." GlobeNewswire, November 3, 2014.

Fang, Lee. "GOP Rep Tom Reed Founded Medical Debt Collection Firm That Harasses His Own Constituents." The Intercept, October 31, 2018.

Farmer, Paul. *Pathologies of Power: Health, Human Rights, and the New War on the Poor*. Berkeley: University of California Press, 2005.

Farmer, Paul. "We Know How to Confront the Coronavirus Pandemic—Expert Mercy." *Boston Globe*, March 19, 2020.

Farmer, Paul. "Who Lives and Who Dies?" *London Review of Books*, February 5, 2015.

"Fifteen Distinguished Alumni Elected to the Drexel 100." *The Drexel 100 Newsletter*, Drexel University Office of Institutional Advancement, Spring 2011.

Finegan, Jay. "48 Hours with the King of Cold Calls." *Inc.*, June 1991.

Fitzgerald, Isaac. *Dirtbag, Massachusetts: A Confessional*. New York: Bloomsbury, 2022.

Friedland, Sandra. "Hospitals Worried About Fund for Poor." *New York Times*, December 23, 1990.

Galbraith, Alison, Dennis Ross-Degnan, Stephen Soumerai, Meredith Rosenthal, Charlene Gay, and Tracy Lieu. "Nearly Half of Families in High-Deductible Health Plans Whose Members Have Chronic Conditions Face Substantial Financial Burden." *Health Affairs* 30, no. 2 (2011): 322–31.

Gale, Arthur. "I Stuffed Their Mouths with Gold: How Hospitals Destroyed the Private Practice of Internal Medicine." *Missouri Medicine* 114, no. 1 (2017): 13–15.

Galloro, Vince. "Making the Best of a Bad (Debt) Situation; Healthcare Organizations Shake Up Their Policies in Light of Increased Scrutiny of Charity Care." *Modern Healthcare*, February 28, 2005.

Gliadkovskaya, Anastassia. "Consumer Financial Protection Bureau Examines Pitfalls in US Medical Billing." Fierce Healthcare, March 3, 2022.

Goff, Robert, and Jerry Ashton. *The Patient, the Doctor, the Bill Collector: A Medical Debt Survival Guide*. Kauai, HI: Hoku House, 2016.

Goldiner, Dave. "State Suspends Medical, Student Debt Collection." *New York Daily News*, March 18, 2020.

Gooch, Kelly. "70% of Americans Trust Their Physicians, 22% Trust Hospital Execs, Survey Finds." *Becker's Hospital Review*, August 10, 2021.

Graeber, David. *Debt: The First 5,000 Years*. New York: Melville House, 2011.

Graeber, David. "Occupy and Anarchism's Gift of Democracy." *The Guardian*, November 15, 2011.

Graeber, David. *The Utopia of Rules: On Technology, Stupidity, and the Secret Joys of Bureaucracy*. New York: Melville House, 2016.

"Grave of Virginia Child AIDS Victim Gets Headstone." *The Washington Post*, June 10, 1985.

Gunderman, Richard. "Medicine and the Pursuit of Wealth." *Hastings Center Report* 28, no. 1 (1998): 9–13.

Halpern, Jake. *Bad Paper: Inside the Secret World of Debt Collectors*. New York: Picador, 2015.

Hancock, Jay, and Elizabeth Lucas. "'UVA Has Ruined Us': Health System Sues Thousands of Patients, Seizing Paychecks and Putting Liens on Homes." *Washington Post*, September 9, 2019.

Hancock, Jay, Elizabeth Lucas, and Kaiser Health News. "UVA Health Revamps Aggressive Debt Collection Practices After Report." *Washington Post*, September 13, 2019.

Hashim, Farah, Sanuri Hennayake, Christi Walsh, Chen Dun, Joseph Giuseppe Paturzo, Indrani G. Das, Emily A. Stewart, et al. "Characteristics of US Hospitals Using Extraordinary Collections Actions Against Patients for Unpaid Medical Bills: A Cross-Sectional Study." *BMJ Open* 12 (2022): e060501.

Haugh, Richard, and Dagmara Scalise. "A Surge in Bad Debt." *Hospitals & Health Networks*, December 2003.

"Hijacker Is Slain; Said Deep in Debt over Medical Bills." *Washington Post*, January 28, 1972.

Himmelstein, David, Deborah Thorne, Elizabeth Warren, and Steffie Woolhandler. "Medical Bankruptcy in the United States: Results of a National Study." *American Journal of Medicine* 122, no. 8 (2009): 741–46.

Himmelstein, David, Elizabeth Warren, Deborah Thorne, and Steffie Woolhandler. "Illness and Injury as Contributors to Bankruptcy." *Health Affairs* 24, S1 (2005): W-5-63–73.

Himmelstein, David, Steffie Woolhandler, Martha Harnly, M. B. Bader, R. Silber, H. D. Backer, and A. A. Jones. "Patient Transfers: Medical Practices as Social Triage." *American Journal of Public Health* 74, no. 5 (1984): 494–97.

Hoffman, Beatrix. "Emergency Rooms: The Reluctant Safety Net." In *History and Health Policy in the United States: Putting the Past Back In*, edited by Rosemary Stevens, Charles Rosenberg, and Lawton Burns, 250–72. New Brunswick, NJ: Rutgers University Press, 2006.

Hoffman, Beatrix. *Health Care for Some: Rights and Rationing in the United States Since 1930*. Chicago: University of Chicago Press, 2012.

Hoffman, Beatrix. "Restraining the Health Care Consumer: Deductibles and Copayments in U.S. Health Insurance." *Social Science History* 30, no. 4 (2006): 501–28.

Holland, Peter. "Junk Justice: A Statistical Study of 4400 Lawsuits Filed by Debt Buyers." *Loyola Consumer Law Review* 26, no. 2 (2014): 179–246.

Holpuch, Amanda. "Medical Debt Is Being Erased in Ohio and Illinois. Is Your Town Next?" *New York Times*, December 29, 2022.

Hyman, Louis. *Debtor Nation: The History of America in Red Ink*. Princeton, NJ: Princeton University Press, 2011.

Iacurci, Greg. "Here's Why Health Savings Accounts Contribute to Inequality." CNBC, April 14, 2022.

Jacoby, Melissa. "The Debtor-Patient Revisited." *Saint Louis University Law Journal* 51, no. 2 (2007): 322–23.

Jacoby, Melissa, and Mirya Holman. "Managing Medical Bills on the Brink of Bankruptcy." *Yale Journal of Health Policy, Law and Ethics* 10, no. 2 (2010): 239–97.

Jacoby, Melissa, and Elizabeth Warren. "Beyond Hospital Misbehavior: An Alternative Account of Medical-Related Financial Distress." *Northwestern University Law Review* 100, no. 2 (2006): 535–84.

"Jeffrey Epsteins's Mentor—Who Once Ran a Ponzi Scheme—Was Found Dead. He was 77." Associated Press, August 26, 2022.

"Jim Richards: A Builder of Business and a Rebuilder of the Collection Industry." Capital Group Radio, March 9, 2016.

Jones, Brian. *Healing Rhode Island: The Story of Rhode Island Hospital, 1863–2013*. East Providence, RI: Signature Printing, 2013.

Jones, Thomas Bard. "Legacy of Change: The Panic of 1819 and Debtor Relief Legislation in the Western States." PhD diss., Cornell University, 1968. ProQuest Dissertations.

Judd, Ron. "ER Doctor Who Criticized Bellingham Hospital's Coronavirus Protections Has Been Fired." *Seattle Times*, March 27, 2020.

Kacik, Alex. "Hospitals' Uncompensated Care Continues to Rise." *Modern Healthcare*, November 21, 2019.

Kalousova, Lucie, and Sarah Burgard. "Debt and Foregone Medical Care." *Journal of Health and Social Behavior* 54, no. 2 (2013): 204–20.

Kane, Nancy, and William Wubbenhorst. "Alternative Funding Policies for the Uninsured: Exploring the Value of Hospital Tax Exemption." *Milbank Quarterly* 78, no. 2 (2000): 185–212.

Kapur, Devesh. "Philanthropy, Self-Interest, and Accountability: American Universities and Developing Countries." In *Giving Well: The Ethics of Philanthropy*, edited by Patricia Illingworth, Thomas Pogge, and Leif Weinar, 264–285. Oxford: Oxford University Press, 2011.

Katz, Michael. *The Price of Citizenship: Redefining the American Welfare State*. Philadelphia: University of Pennsylvania Press, 2008.

Kennedy, Edward M. *In Critical Condition: The Crisis in America's Health Care*. New York: Simon & Schuster, 1971.

Kennedy, John W. "US Navy Vet/Social Entrepreneur Jerry Ashton Says End Veteran Medical Debt." Let's Rethink This, March 7, 2022.

Kiel, Paul, and Jeff Ernthausen. "Debt Collectors Have Made a Fortune This Year. Now They're Coming for More." ProPublica, October 5, 2020.

Klemm, John. "Medicaid Spending: A Brief History." *Health Care Financing Review* 22, no. 1 (2000): 105–12.

Sarah Kliff. "The Doctor's Strike That Nearly Killed Canada's Medicare-for-all Plan, Explained." *Vox*, March 29, 2019.

Kliff, Sarah. "With Medical Bills Skyrocketing, More Hospitals Are Suing for Payment." *New York Times*, November 8, 2019.

Kliff, Sarah. "Why I'm Obsessed with Patients' Medical Bills." *New York Times*, August 7, 2020.

Klozotsky, Michael. "How a (Non-Apple) U.S. Patent Might Just Change the World." *Forbes*, July 31, 2012.

Kluender, Raymond, Neale Mahoney, Francis Wong, and Wesley Yin. "Medical Debt in the US, 2009–2020." *Journal of the American Medical Association* 326, no. 3 (2021): 250–56.

Kodjak, Alison. "Widowed Early, a Cancer Doctor Writes About the Harm of Medical Debt." NPR, August 10, 2017.

Kosman, Josh. *The Buyout of America: How Private Equity Is Killing Jobs and Destroying the American Economy*. New York: Portfolio, 2010.

Kovac, Susan. "Judgment-Proof Debtors in Bankruptcy." *American Bankruptcy Law Journal* 65, no. 5 (1991): 681.

Krugman, Paul. "Don't Make Health Care a Purity Test." *New York Times*, March 21, 2019.

Kutscher, Bert. "Medical Debt Collectors Frustrated by FCC Cellphone Ruling." *Modern Healthcare*, August 29, 2015.

Lagnado, Lucette. "Call It Yale v. Yale: Law-School Clinic Is Taking Affiliated Hospital to Court over Debt Collection Tactics." *Wall Street Journal*, November 14, 2003.

Lagnado, Lucette. "Hospitals Try Extreme Measures to Collect Their Overdue Debts: Patients Who Skip Hearings." *Wall Street Journal*, October 30, 2003.

Lagnado, Lucette. "Jeanette White Is Long Dead but Her Hospital Bill Lives On." *Wall Street Journal*, March 13, 2003.

Lagnado, Lucette. "Twenty Years—and He Isn't Paying Any More." *Wall Street Journal*, April 1, 2003.

Lando, Tamar. "Pocket Protector: KB Forbes Is Defending Uninsured Patients. Never Mind Why." *Mother Jones*, May/June 2005.

Last Week Tonight with John Oliver, Season 3, Episode 14, "Debt Buyers," HBO, June 5, 2016. https://www.youtube.com/watch?v=hxUAntt1z2c

Lee, Chulho Christopher. "The Financial Impacts of Bad Debt in the Healthcare Industry: A Multivariate Statistical Analysis." PhD diss., St. Louis University, 1996.

Lefton, Ray. "Developing Organizational Charity-Care Policies and Procedures." *Healthcare Financial Management* 56, no. 4 (2002): 52–57.

Lefton, Ray. "What's It Worth? Cost Shifting, a Practice That Can Often Result in Significant Financial Burden on Self-Pay Patients, Is Leading to Greater Scrutiny of Hospital Charging Practices." *Healthcare Financial Management* 57, no. 12 (2003): 60.

Levey, Noam. "Investigation: Many US Hospitals Sue Patients for Debts or Threaten Their Credit." NPR, December 21, 2022.

Levey, Noam. "Sick and Struggling to Pay, 100 Million People in the U.S. Live with Medical Debt." NPR, June 16, 2022.

Lewis, Larry. "Big Collections from Little Debt Debts Have a Montco Firm Growing." *Philadelphia Inquirer*, January 16, 1992.

Limpe, Michelle. "Protesters Advocate for Legislation to Alleviate Burden of Medical Debt Lawsuits." *The Johns Hopkins News-Letter*, April 10, 2021.

Liss, Samantha. "When a Nonprofit Health System Outsources Its ER, Debt Collectors Follow." *St. Louis Post-Dispatch*, April 17, 2016.

Locker, Kitty O. "'Sir, This Will Never Do': Model Dunning Letters, 1592–1873." *Journal of Business Communication* 22, no. 2 (1973): 39–45.

Lunsford, Patrick. "NCO Settles Debt Collection Action with 19 States." InsideARM, February 7, 2012.

Luthra, Shefali. "Bank Loans Signed in the Hospital Leave Patients Vulnerable." *Los Angeles Times*, February 21, 2018.

Magnus, Stephen Alexander. "Agency Implications of Debt in Not-for-Profit Hospitals." PhD diss., University of Michigan, 2002.

Makary, Marty. *The Price We Pay: What Broke American Healthcare and How to Fix It.* New York: Bloomsbury, 2019.

Marino, Vivian. "Debt Collectors Thrive as Borrowers Binge." *Las Vegas Review*, April 15, 1996.

Martino, Amy. "Tricap Technology Group's CEO Refuses to Wait for Opportunity to Knock." *Sync*, August 12, 2016.

"Maryland Healthcare Collection Bill Becomes Law." Accountsrecovery.net, June 8, 2021.

"Medical Debt Policy Scorecard." Innovation for Justice, University of Arizona and University of Utah. Accessed December 10, 2022. https://medicaldebtpolicysc orecard.org

"Medical Debt Turning into Credit Card Debt." *St. Louis Post-Dispatch*, June 11, 2008.

Mencarini, Matt. "Medical Debt Collection Continues Amid Pandemic." *Cincinnati Enquirer*, July 24, 2020.

Messac, Luke. "Lifespan, Stop Suing My Patients." *UpriseRI*, September 19, 2019.

Michas, Frederic. "Number of Hospitals in the U.S., 1975–2019." *Statista*, February 9, 2021.

Michigan Law Review Editorial Board. "The Unnecessary Doctrine of Necessaries." *Michigan Law Review* 82, no. 7 (1984): 1767–99.

Moon, Josh. "Who Is KB Forbes? The Answer Isn't Hard to Find or All That Unexpected." *Alabama Political Reporter*, July 16, 2020.

Mulstein, Suzanne. "The Uninsured and the Financing of Uncompensated Care: Scope, Costs and Policy Options." *Inquiry* 21, no. 3 (1984): 214–29.

Murphy, Andrea. "America's Largest Private Companies: Cargill Is Back at No. 1." *Forbes*, November 23, 2021.

Murphy, Tom. "Health Care Company Grows by Piling Up Debt: After Six Years, Senex Services Corp. Expands Its Collection Business in a Field That Is Ripe for Growth." *Indianapolis Business Journal* 24, no. 53 (2004): 9.

Natarajan, Prabha. "No Grass Under These Young Feet: Three CEOs Strike Gold Before 40." *Philadelphia Business Journal*, August 2, 1999. https://www.bizjournals. com/philadelphia/stories/1999/08/02/focus2.html.

Nemes, Judith. "Hospitals Put Teeth into Efforts to Collect Bad Debt." *Modern Healthcare* 21, no. 24 (1991): 41–50.

Nichols, John. "Obama's 'Eager to See' Better Approach on Health Reform." *The Nation,* January 28, 2010.

Nova, Annie. "She's Been Pushing for Student Loan Forgiveness for a Decade. Now It Could Happen." CNBC, May 15, 2022.

Oberlander, Jonathan. *The Political Life of Medicare*. Chicago: University of Chicago Press, 2003.

O'Brien, Dennis. "Hospitals Sue to Collect from Uninsured Patients." *Baltimore Sun*, August 15, 1993.

O'Farrell, Peggy. "Seeking a Cure for Medical Debt." *Cincinnati Enquirer*, May 4, 2008.

Oppenheimer, Mark. "Oppenheimer on the Advocate." *New Haven Review*, December 3, 2013.

Orwell, George. *Down and Out in Paris and London.* Morrisville, NC: Lulu Press, 2012 (1933).

Orwell, George. "Politics and the English Language." In *A Collection of Essays*, 156–70. Orlando, FL: Harvest, 1981.

O'Toole, Thomas, Jose Arbelaez, and Bruce Dixon. "Full Disclosure of Financial Costs and Options to Patients: The Roles of Race, Age, Health Insurance, and Usual Source for Care." *Journal of Healthcare for the Poor and Underserved* 15, no. 1 (2004): 52–62.

O'Toole, Thomas, Jose Arbalaez, and Robert Lawrence. "Medical Debt and Aggressive Debt Restitution Practices." *Journal of General Internal Medicine* 19 (2004): 772–78.

Otremba, Michael, Gretchen Berland, and Joseph Amon. "Hospitals as Debtor Prisons." *Lancet Global Health* 3, no. 5 (2015): e253–54.

Owens, Caitlin. "America's Biggest Hospitals vs. Their Patients." Axios, June 14, 2021.

Paavola, Alia. "Maryland Changes Medical Debt Collection Rules for Hospitals." *Becker's Hospital Review*, January 4, 2022.

Packer, George. *The Unwinding: An Inner History of America*. New York: Farrar, Straus & Giroux, 2013.

Peebles, Gustav. "Washing Away the Sins of Debt: The Nineteenth-Century Eradication of the Debtors' Prison." *Comparative Studies in Society and History* 55, no. 3 (2013): 701–14.

Pell, M. P. "Patients in Arrears Face Collectors: Agencies Buy Up Delinquent Accounts." *Atlanta Journal-Constitution*, June 5, 2011: B1.

Piola, Chuck. *Going in Cold: How to Turn Strangers into Clients and Get Rich Doing It*. Washington, DC: Folger Ross, 2005.

Pisu, Maria, Nora Hendrikson, Matthew Banegas, and K. Robin Yabroff. "Costs of Cancer Along the Care Continuum: What We Can Expect Based on Recent Literature." *Cancer* 124, no. 21 (2018): 4181–91.

Pope Francis. *Angelus*. Gemelli University Hospital, Rome, Italy, July 11, 2021.

Potts, Gregory. "Surprising Rewards in Debt Collection." *Journal Record (Oklahoma City)*, September 13, 1999.

Regula, Ralph. "National Policy and the Medically Uninsured." *Inquiry* 24, no. 1 (1987): 48–56.

Rice, Thomas, Wilm Quentin, Anders Anell, Andrew J. Barnes, Pauline Rosenau, Lynn Y. Unruh, and Ewout van Ginnekin. "Revisiting Out-of-Pocket Requirements: Trends in Spending, Financial Access Barriers, and Policy in Ten High-Income Countries." *BMC Health Services Research* 18, no. 18 (2018): 371.

Richards, Leonard. *Shays Rebellion: The American Revolution's Final Battle*. Philadelphia: University of Pennsylvania Press, 2003.

Robertson, Christopher, Mark Rukavina, and Erin Fuse Brown. "New State Consumer Protections Against Medical Debt." *Journal of the American Medical Association* 327, no. 2 (2022): 121–22.

Rosen, George. *Fees and Fee Bills: Some Economic Aspects of Medical Practice in Nineteenth Century America*. Baltimore: Johns Hopkins University Press, 1946.

Rosenberg, Charles. *The Care of Strangers: The Rise of America's Hospital System*. New York: Basic Books, 1987.

Rosenberg, Hannah. "It Is Hard to Let Your Heart Break." Unpublished poem, 2022.

Rosenthal, Brian. "One Hospital System Sued 2500 Patients After Pandemic Hit." *New York Times*, January 5, 2021.

Rosner, David. *A Once Charitable Enterprise: Hospitals and Health Care in Brooklyn and New York, 1885–1915*. New York: Cambridge University Press, 1982.

Ross, Andrew, and Astra Taylor. "Rolling Jubilee Is a Spark—Not the Solution." *The Nation*, November 27, 2012.

Rowan, Lisa. "70% of Medical Collection Debt Will Soon Be Removed from Credit Reports: Here's What You Need to Know." *Forbes*, April 5, 2022.

Sanders, Linley. "Comparing American and British Attitudes on Health Care in 2022." YouGov, October 24, 2022.

Sanger-Katz, Margot, Julie Creswell, and Reed Abelson. "Mystery Solved: Private-Equity Backed Firms Are Behind Ad Blitz on 'Surprise Billing.'" *New York Times*, September 30, 2021.

Santini, Maureen. "Mondale Says Reagan 'Out of Step with America.'" Associated Press, August 14, 1980.

Saywell, Robert, Terrell Zollinger, David Chu, C. A. Macbeth, and M. E. Sechrist. "Hospital and Patient Characteristics of Uncompensated Hospital Care: Policy Implications." *Journal of Health Politics, Policy and Law* 14, no. 2 (1989): 287–307.

Schorr, Daniel. *Don't Get Sick in America*. Chicago: Aurora, 1970.

Scott, Lisa. "Firm Offers to Sell Bad Debt to Highest Bidder." *Modern Healthcare*, February 8, 1993.

Seifert, Robert. "The Demand Side of Financial Exploitation: The Case of Medical Debt." *Housing Policy Debate* 15, no. 3 (2010): 785–803.

Seifert, Robert, and Mark Rukavina. "Bankruptcy Is the Tip of a Medical-Debt Iceberg." *Health Affairs* 25, no. 2 (2006): W89–92.

Sherlock, Douglas. "Indigent Care in Rational Markets." *Inquiry* 23, no. 3 (1986): 261–67.

Shi, Leiyu, and Douglas Singh. *Delivering Health Care in America: A Systems Approach*. 7th ed. Burlington: MA: Jones & Bartlett, 2017.

Shinkman, Ron. "An Interview with K. B. Forbes, Advocate for the Uninsured." Fierce Healthcare, January 19, 2015.

Shultz, Blake, Alexander Janke, and Arjun Venkatesh. "Hospital Debt Collection Practices Require Urgent Reform." *Health Affairs Forefront*, May 2, 2022.

Silver-Greenberg, Jessica, and Katie Thomas. "They Were Entitled to Free Care. Hospitals Hounded Them to Pay." *New York Times*, September 24, 2022.

Simmons-Duffin, Selena. "When Hospitals Sue for Unpaid Bills, It Can Be 'Ruinous' for Patients." NPR, June 25, 2019.

Sloan, Allan. "The SEC vs Steven Hoffenberg: A Case of Leaning Fortunes at Towers Financial?" *Washington Post*, February 16, 1993.

Starr, Paul. *The Social Transformation of American Medicine: The Rise of a Sovereign Profession and the Making of a Vast Industry*. New York: Basic Books, 1982.

Stevens, Rosemary. *In Sickness and in Wealth: American Hospitals in the Twentieth Century*. Baltimore: Johns Hopkins University Press, 1999.

"Stirrings in Medical Debt." *Collections & Credit Risk* 5, no. 7 (2000): 18.

Sullivan, Teresa, Elizabeth Warren, and Jay Westbrook. *The Fragile Middle Class: Americans in Debt*. New Haven, CT: Yale University Press, 2000.

Sullivan, Teresa, Jay Lawrence Westbrook, and Elizabeth Warren. *As We Forgive Our Debtors: Bankruptcy and Consumer Credit in America*. Fairless Hills, PA: Beard Books, 1999.

Taylor, Astra. "From the Ashes of Occupy: On Failing Better and Erasing Debts." *Hazlitt*, November 14, 2013.

Taylor, Astra. *Remake the World: Essays, Reflections, Rebellions*. Chicago: Haymarket Books, 2021.

Taylor, John J. *The Physician as a Business Man; Or, How to Obtain the Best Financial Results in the Practice of Medicine*. Philadelphia: The Medical World, 1892.

Taylor, Mar. "Full-Court Press." *Modern Healthcare* 34 (2004): 32–33.

Tek Sehgal, Raj, and Paul Gorman. "Internal Medicine Physicians' Knowledge of Health Care Charges." *Journal of Graduate Medical Education* 3, no. 2 (2011): 182–87.

Thomas, Wendi. "A Tennessee Hospital Sues Its Own Employees When They Can't Pay Their Medical Bills." NPR, June 28, 2019.

Thomas, Wendi. "This Doctors Group Is Owned by a Private Equity Firm and Repeatedly Sued the Poor Until We Called Them." ProPublica, November 27, 2019.

Thornton, Tamara Plaikins. "'A Great Machine' or a 'Beast of Prey': A Boston Corporation and Its Rural Debtors in an Age of Capitalist Transformation." *Journal of the Early American Republic* 27, no. 4 (2007): 567–97.

"Tom Gores." *Forbes*, accessed July 15, 2022, https://www.forbes.com/profile/tom-gores/?sh=2804e2ab6b39

Tomes, Nancy. *Remaking the American Patient: How Madison Avenue and Modern Medicine Turned Patients into Consumers*. Chapel Hill: University of North Carolina Press, 2016.

"Transworld Systems Signs Agreement with AMA to Provide Accounts Receivable Management Solutions to Member Physicians." InsideARM, March 7, 2011.

Traub, Amy. "Credit Reports and Employment: Findings from the 2012 National Survey on Credit Card Debt of Low- and Middle-Income Households." *Suffolk University Law Review* 46 (2013): 983–95.

Tumulty, Brian. "Reed Answers Ethics Questions." *Democrat & Chronicle*, February 24, 2014.

Tzu, Sun. *The Art of War*. Trans. Lionel Giles. New York: Dover, 2002.

Unger, Harlow Giles. *John Quincy Adams*. New York: Hachette, 2012.

Villagra, Victor, Mario Felix, Emil Coman, Denise O. Smith, Allison Joslyn, Trisha Pitter, and Wizdom Powell. "When Hospitals and Doctors Sue Their Patients: The Medical Debt Crisis Through a New Lens." Health Disparities Institute Issue Brief, June 2019.

Wang, Yang, Ge Bai, and Gerard Anderson. "COVID-19 and Hospital Financial Viability in the US." *JAMA Health Forum* 3, no. 5 (2022): e221018.

Warren, Elizabeth. "Sick and Broke." *Washington Post*, February 9, 2005.

Warren, Elizabeth, and Amelia Warren Tyagi. *The Two-Income Trap: Why Middle-Class Parents Are Going Broke*. New York: Basic Books, 2004.

Webster, Charles. "Note on 'Stuffing their Mouths with Gold'." In *Aneurin Bevan on the National Health Service*, 219–22. Oxford: Wellcome Unit for the History of Medicine, 1991.

Weissman, Joel, Carol van Deusen Lukas, and Arnold Epstein. "Bad Debt and Free Care in Massachusetts Hospitals." *Health Affairs* 11, no. 2 (1992): 148–61.

Weissmann, Dan. "A Legendary Lawyer Sued Hospitals for Price-Gouging Their Patients. And Got His Butt Handed to Him." *An Arm and a Leg* podcast, Season 6, Episode 2, September 2, 2021. https://armandalegshow.com/episode/a-legendary-lawyer-sued-hospitals-for-price-gouging-their-patients-and-got-his-butt-handed-to-him

Weissmann, Dan. "Viral TikTok Video Serves Up Recipe to 'Crush' Medical Debt." *An Arm and a Leg* podcast, Season 4, Episode 16, February 15, 2021. https://armandalegshow.com/episode/dollar-for

Wilde Mathews, Anna, Andrea Fuller, and Melanie Evans. "Hospitals Often Don't Help Needy Patients, Even Those Who Qualify." *Wall Street Journal*, November 17, 2022.

Wilkes, Michael, and David Schriger. "Why Won't UC Clinics Serve Patients with State-Funded Health Insurance?" *Los Angeles Times*, April 4, 2022.

Wilson, Cynthia. "Health Care Receivables Pose More Challenges Than Opportunities for Big Debt Collectors." InsideARM, March 7, 2011.

Winkour Munk, Cheryl. "New Debt-Collection Rules: What they Mean for Consumers." *Wall Street Journal*, January 7, 2022.

Wolf, Jeff, and Mike Passanante. "Medicare Bad Debt 101." *The Hospital Finance Podcast*, May 25, 2022. https://www.besler.com/insights/medicare-bad-debt-101

"Worried by Debt, He Tries Suicide." *Atlanta Journal-Constitution*, October 10, 1912.

Wu, Chi Chi. "Medical Debt." *Clearinghouse Review Journal of Poverty Law and Policy* 39, nos. 7–8 (2005): 465–85.

Xu, Ke, David Evans, Guido Carrin, Ana Mylena Aguilar-Rivera, Philip Musgrove, and Timothy Evans. "Protecting Households from Catastrophic Health Spending." *Health Affairs* 26, no. 4 (2007): 972–83.

Yabroff, K. Robin, Jingxuan Zhao, Xuesong Han, and Zhiyuan Zheng. "Prevalence and Correlates of Medical Financial Hardship in the USA." *Journal of General Internal Medicine* 34, no. 8 (2019): 1494–1502.

Yerak, Becky. "Medical Debt Collection, Reporting Under Scrutiny." *Chicago Tribune*, December 11, 2014.

Zadoorian, James, Thomas Bernardin, and Ashley Hodgson. "Patient-Centric Aid in a Consumer-Driven Marketplace." *Healthcare Financial Management*, December 1, 2018.

Zremski, Jerry. "Reed's Law Firm Operated Under His Name." *Buffalo News*, February 22, 2014.

INDEX

For the benefit of digital users, indexed terms that span two pages (e.g., 52–53) may, on occasion, appear on only one of those pages.